Lip-reading Puzzles (1)

by Tony Edens

2018

Also in this series:

Lip Reading a self-help textbook

The Lip Reading Dictionary

The Lip Reading Thesaurus
of 3000 look alike words

The Lip Readers' Picture Book of
misheard phrases

Introduction

Most people lip-read a bit though they don't know it. We probably obtained this skill at a very young age as we learned to speak and to interpret the speech of our mother. As time went by we began to rely more upon what we heard and less on what we could lip-read. So lip-reading was pushed to the background only to be used in very noisy situations when we couldn't hear properly. We all have the skill – its just that we don't use it very often, and when we do we are not usually aware that we are doing it.

The puzzles in this book are intended to to help us to re-awaken our hidden ability to lip-read so that it can be available for us to use as our hearing deteriorates over the years.

The puzzles concentrate only on the initial sound of the words or phrases used – but the principles are the same whether the sounds are at the start, middle or end of words.

Puzzles 1 to 10 contain only words that use the basic lip-shapes as illustrated in section 51.

Puzzles 11 to 50 contain a wider set of lip-shapes in which some of the lip shapes have been modified by another sound that precedes or follows it. More information about modified lip-shapes is given in section 52.

Contents

Lip-reading puzzle:

1. supermarket

The pictures below represent things found in a **supermarket** as a spoken list. The lip shape shown for each is the first seen by a lip-reader.

Here are the words as a written list:
Early potatoes, sugar, lettuce, bananas, ravioli, navel oranges, thick cut loaf, frozen peas, yoghurt, winter cabbage

Can you match the words on the list to the correct lip-shapes?

1.__________

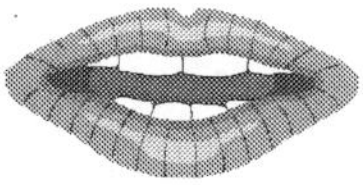

2.__________

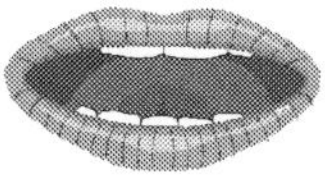

3.__________

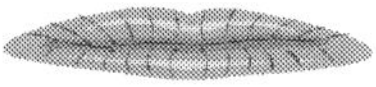

4.__________

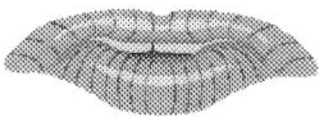

5.__________

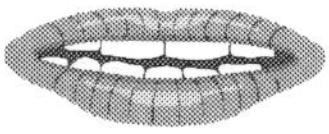

6.__________

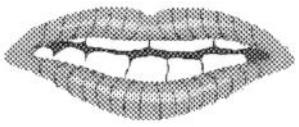

7.__________

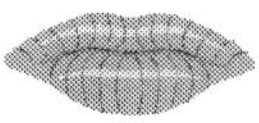

8.__________

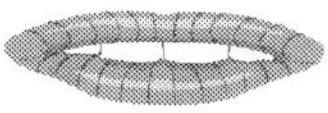

9.__________

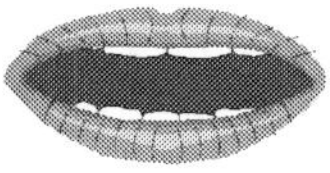

10.__________

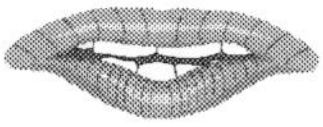

Solution:

1. supermarket

puzzle

The written list was:

Early potatoes, sugar, lettuce, bananas, ravioli, navel oranges, thick cut loaf, frozen peas, yoghurt, winter cabbage

The words can be matched to their respective initial lip-shapes in the following order.

1.
thick cut loaf

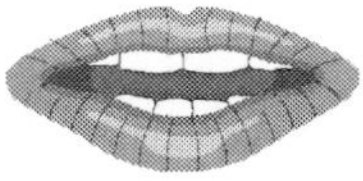

2.
lettuce

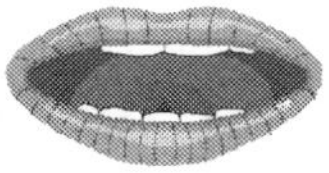

3.
bananas

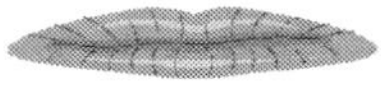

4.
ravioli

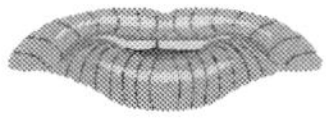

5.
navel oranges

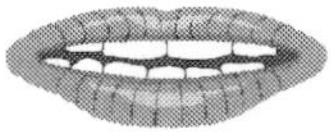

6.
yoghurt

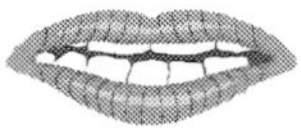

7.
winter cabbage

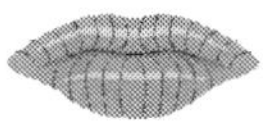

8.
frozen peas

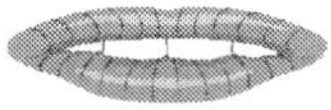

9.
early potatoes

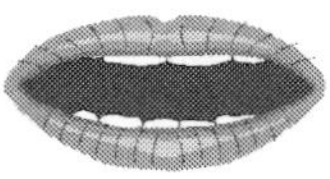

10.
sugar

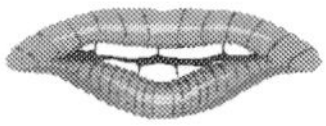

Lip-reading puzzle:

2. things to eat

The pictures below represent **things to eat** as a spoken list. The lip shape shown for each is the first that would be seen by a lip-reader

Here are the words as a written list:
Arctic roll, Eve's pudding, juice, lemon pie, pancake, omelette, rissole, Upside-down cake, water biscuit, flapjack.

Can you match the words on the list to the correct lip-shapes?

1.__________

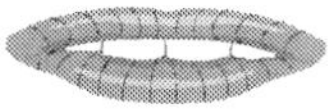

2.__________

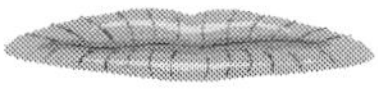

3.__________

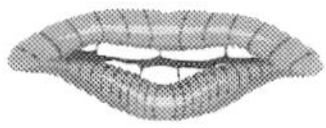

4.__________

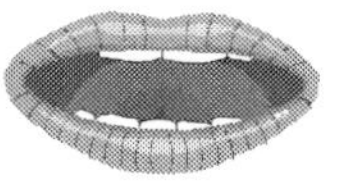

5.__________

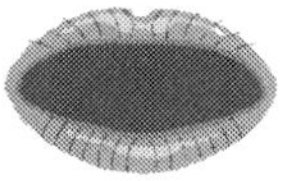

6.__________

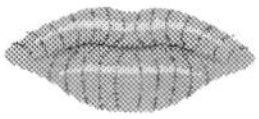

7.__________

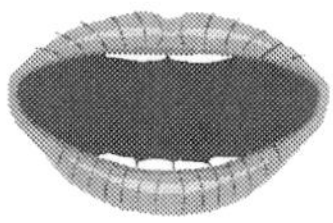

8.__________

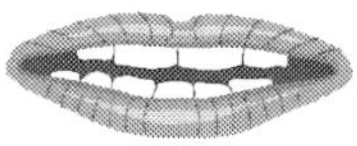

9.__________

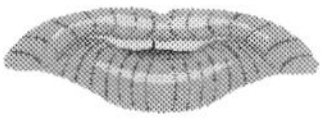

10.__________

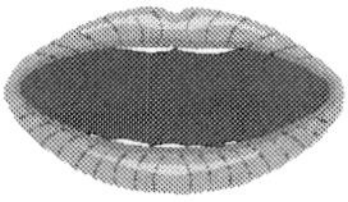

Solution:

2. things to eat

puzzle

The written list was:

Arctic roll, Eve's pudding, juice, lemon pie, pancake, omelette, rissole, Upside-down cake, water biscuit, flapjack.

The words can be matched to their respective initial lip-shapes in the following order.

1. flapjack

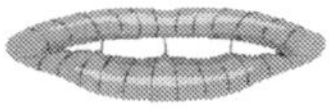

2. pancake

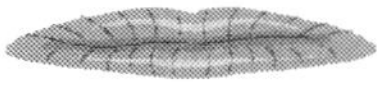

3. juice

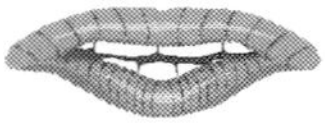

4. lemon pie

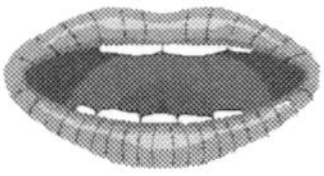

5. omelette

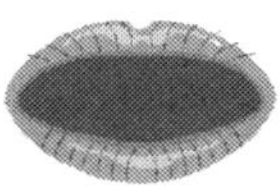

6. water biscuit

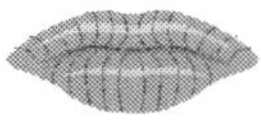

7. arctic roll

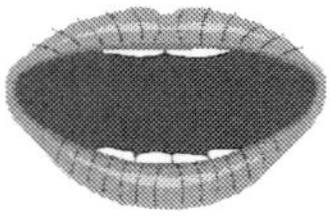

8. Eve's pudding

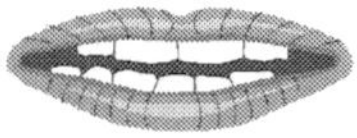

9. rissole

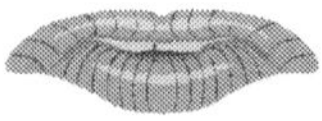

10. Upside-down cake

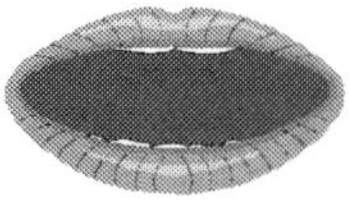

Lip-reading puzzle:

3. ways to travel

The pictures below represent **ways to travel** as a spoken list. The lip shape shown for each word is the first lip shape that would be seen by a lip-reader as the word is spoken.

Here are the words as a written list:
Amble, inch, jump, linger, breast stroke, run, dive, fly, walk.

Can you match the words on the list to the correct lip-shapes?

1.__________

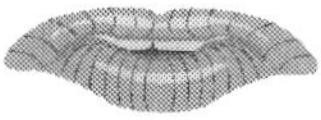

2.__________

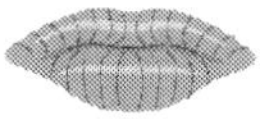

3.__________

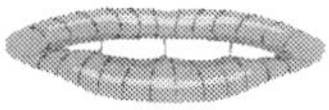

4.__________

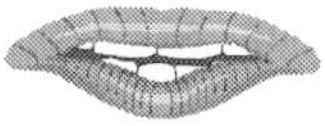

5.__________

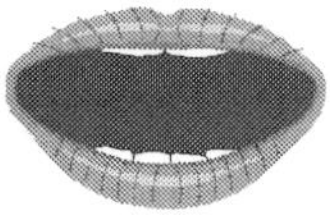

6.__________

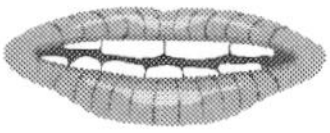

7.__________

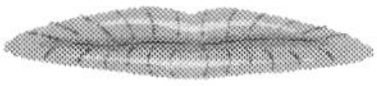

8.__________

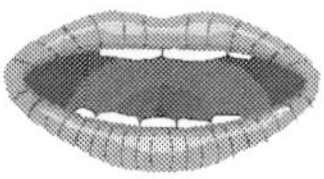

9.__________.

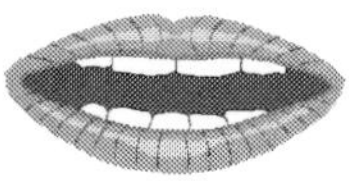

Solution:

3. ways to travel

puzzle

The written list was:

Amble, inch, jump, linger, breast stroke, run, dive, fly, walk.

The words can be matched to their respective initial lip-shapes in the following order.

1.
run

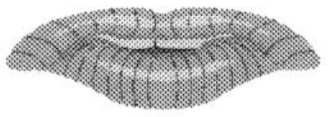

2.
walk

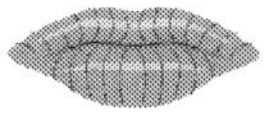

3.
fly

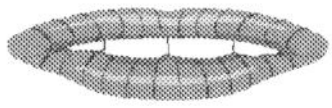

4.
jump

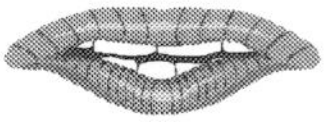

5.
amble

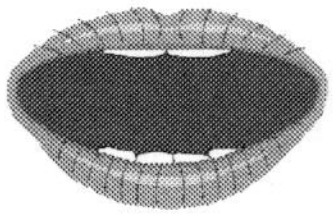

6.
dive

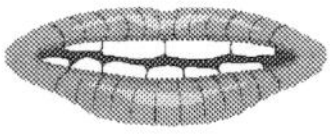

7.
breast stroke

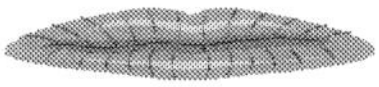

8.
linger

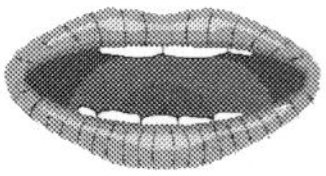

9.
inch

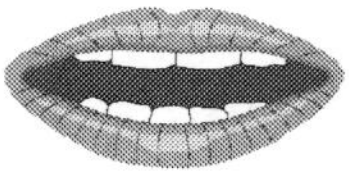

Lip-reading puzzle:

4. bus travel

The pictures below represent words connected with **bus travel** as a spoken list. The lip shape shown for each word is the first lip shape that would be seen by a lip-reader as the word is spoken.

Here are the words as a written list:
Adults, inside, children, passengers, omnibus, route, driver, fare, windows, used tickets.

Can you match the words on the list to the correct lip-shapes?

1.__________

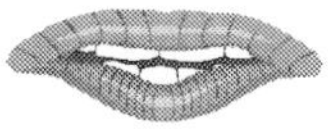

2.__________

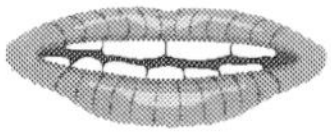

3.__________

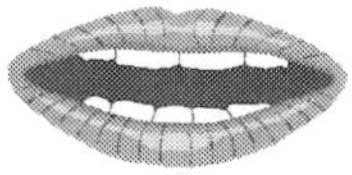

4.__________

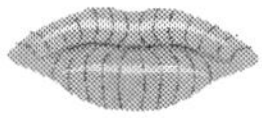

5.__________

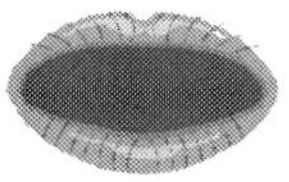

6.__________

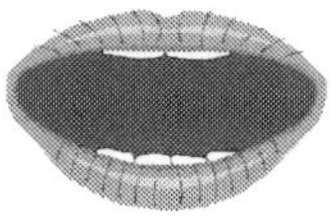

7.__________

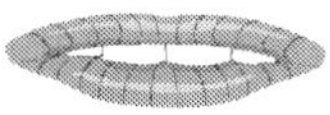

8.__________

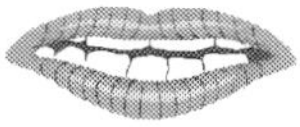

9.__________

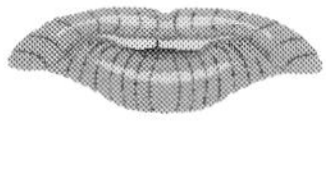

10.__________

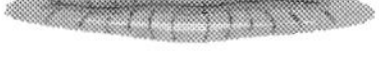

Solution:

4. bus travel

puzzle

The written list was:

Adults, inside, children, passengers, omnibus, route, driver, fare, windows, used tickets.

The words can be matched to their respective initial lip-shapes in the following order.

1. children

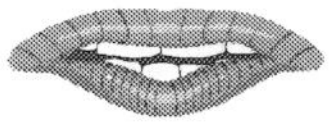

2. driver

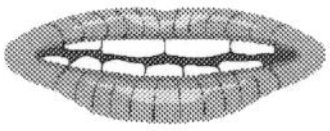

3. inside

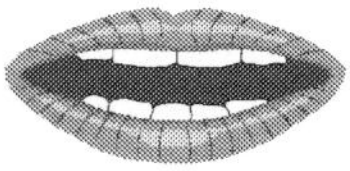

4. windows

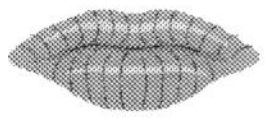

5. omnibus

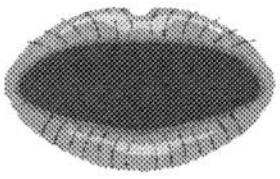

6. adults

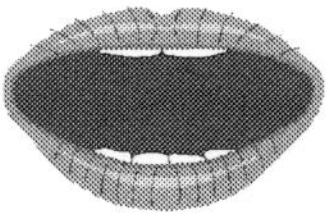

7. fare

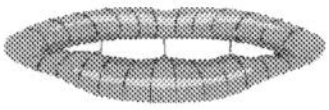

8. used tickets

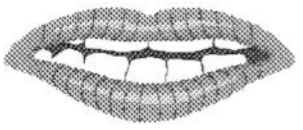

9. route

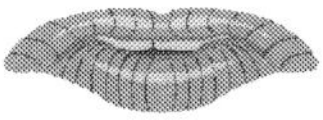

10. passengers

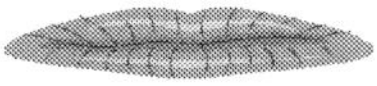

Lip-reading puzzle:

5. church

The pictures below represent things or people in a **church** as a spoken list. The lip shape shown for each word is the first lip shape that would be seen by a lip-reader as the word is spoken.

Here are the words as a written list:
Altar, incense, aisle, chancel, lights, minister, robes, stained glass, font, warden.

Can you match the words on the list to the correct lip-shapes?

1.__________ 2.__________ 3.__________ 4.__________

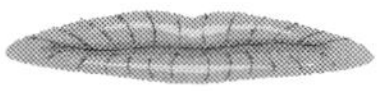 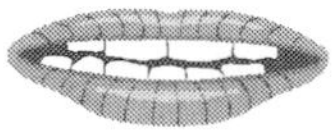 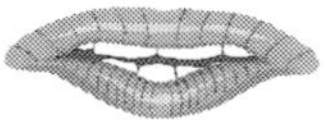 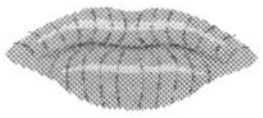

5.__________ 6.__________ 7.__________ 8.__________

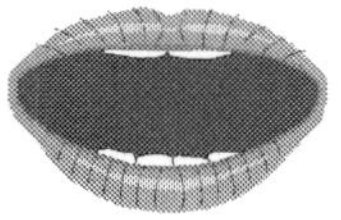 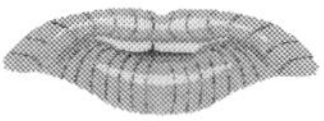 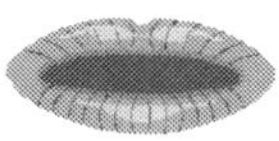 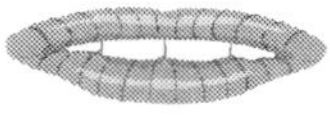

9.__________ 10.__________

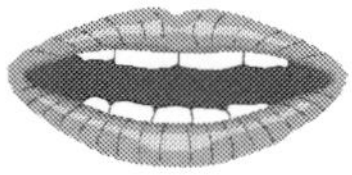 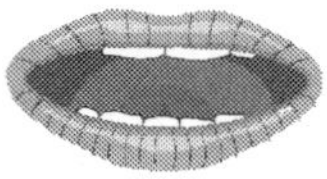

Solution:

5. church

puzzle

The written list was:

Altar, incense, aisle, chancel, lights, minister, robes, stained glass, font, warden.

The words can be matched to their respective initial lip-shapes in the following order.

1. minister

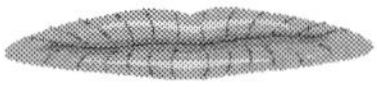

2. stained glass

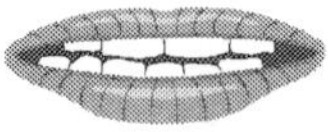

3. chancel

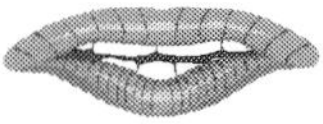

4. warden

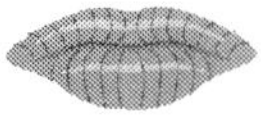

5. aisle

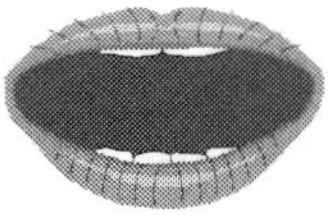

6. robes

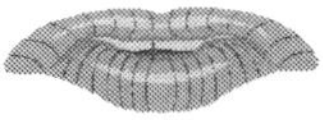

7. altar

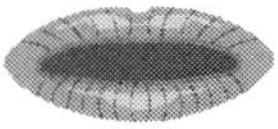

8. font

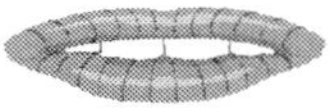

9. incense

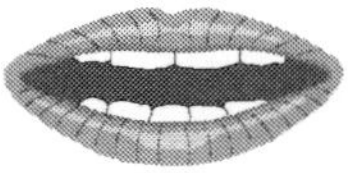

10. lights

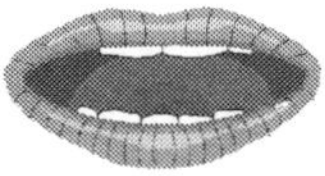

Lip-reading puzzle:

6. houses

The pictures below represent words to do with **houses** as a spoken list. The lip shape shown for each is the first that would be seen by a lip-reader.

Here are the words as a written list:
Entrance, chimney, letterbox, bathroom, roof, door, thatch, French window, utilities room, bathroom.

Can you match the words on the list to the correct lip-shapes?

1.__________ 2.__________ 3.__________ 4.__________

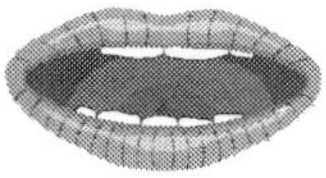 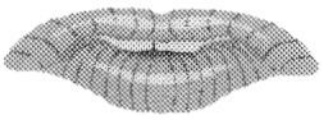 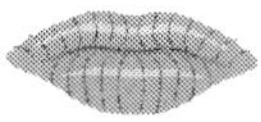 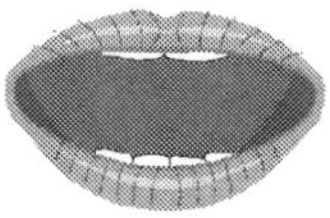

5.__________ 6.__________ 7.__________ 8.__________

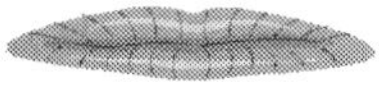 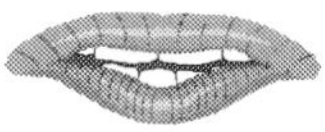 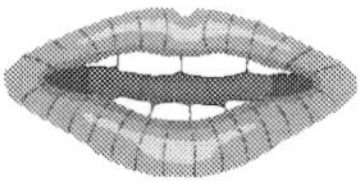 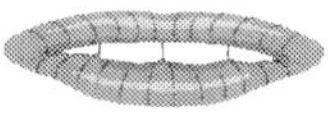

9.__________ 10.__________

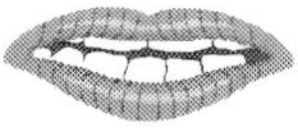 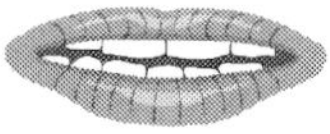

Solution:

6. houses

puzzle

The written list was:

Entrance, chimney, letterbox, bathroom, roof, door, thatch, French window, utilities room, bathroom.

The words can be matched to their respective initial lip-shapes in the following order.

1. letterbox

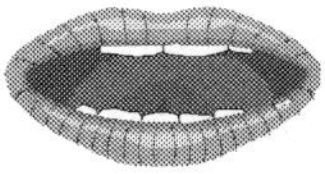

2. roof

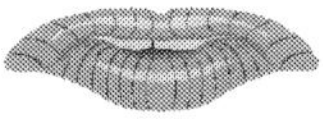

3. window

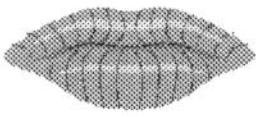

4. entrance

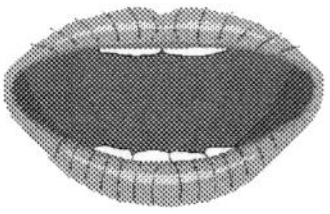

5. bathroom

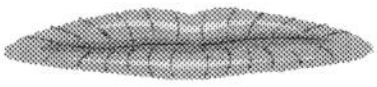

6. chimney

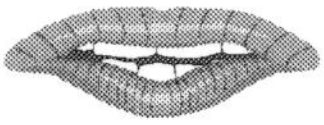

7. thatch

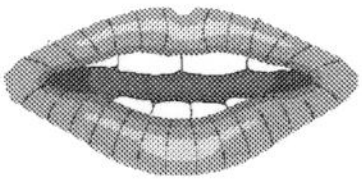

8. French window

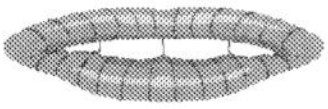

9. utilities room

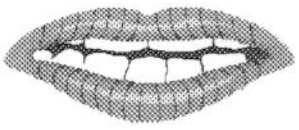

10. door

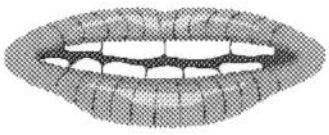

Lip-reading puzzle:

7. nature

The pictures below represent words to do with **nature** as a spoken list. The lip shape shown for each word is the first lip shape that would be seen by a lip-reader as the word is spoken.

Here are the words as a written list:
Antelope, elephant, emu, urchin, ladybird, otter, rabbit, thistle, fish, whale.

Can you match the words on the list to the correct lip-shapes?

1.__________

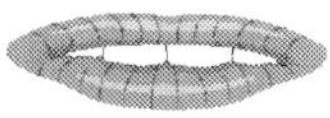

2.__________

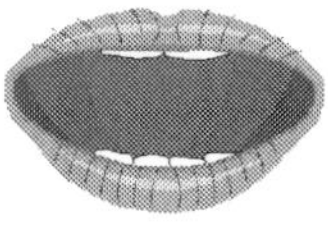

3.__________

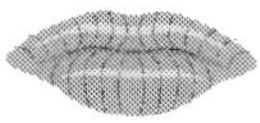

4.__________

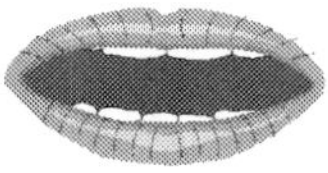

5.__________

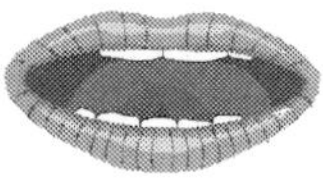

6.__________

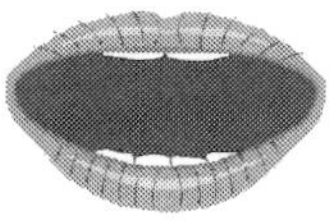

7.__________

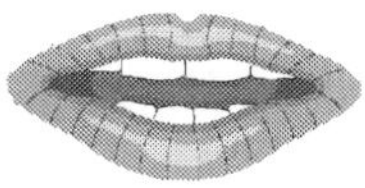

8.__________

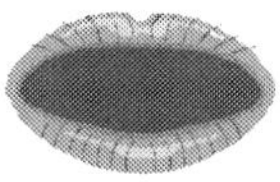

9.__________

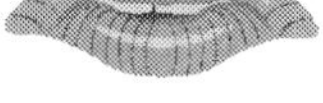

10.__________

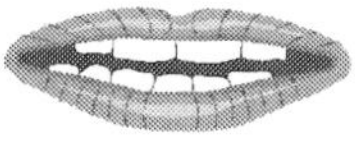

Solution:

7. nature

puzzle

The written list was:

Antelope, elephant, emu, urchin, ladybird, otter, rabbit, thistle, fish, whale.

whale The words can be matched to their respective initial lip-shapes in the following order.

1. fish

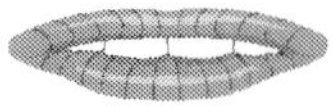

2. elephant

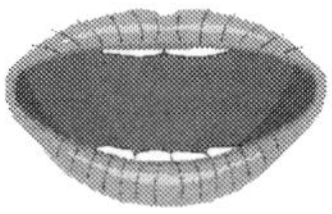

3. whale

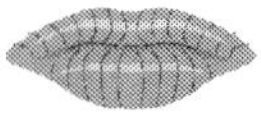

4. urchin

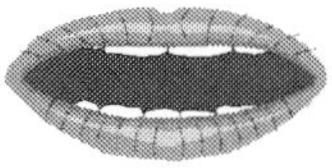

5. ladybird

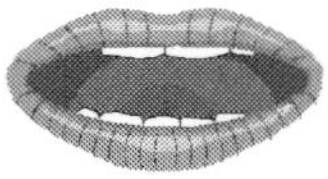

6. antelope

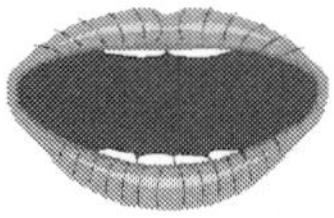

7. thistle

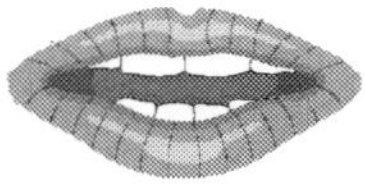

8. otter

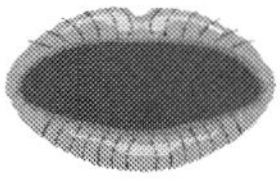

9. rabbit

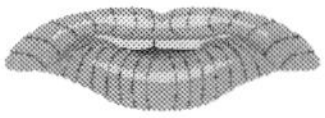

10. emu

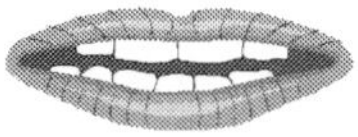

Lip-reading puzzle:

8. plants

The pictures below represent words to do with **plants** as a spoken list. The lip shape shown for each word is the first lip shape that would be seen by a lip-reader as the word is spoken.

Here are the words as a written list:
Anthers, inner leaf, shoot, leaf, petal, ovary, root, stem, flower, wilting.

Can you match the words on the list to the correct lip-shapes?

1.__________ 2.__________ 3.__________ 4.__________

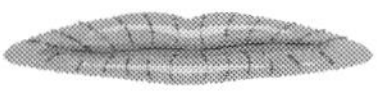
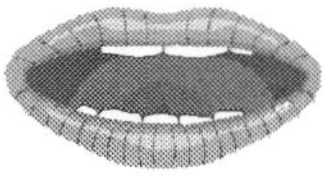
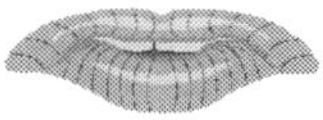
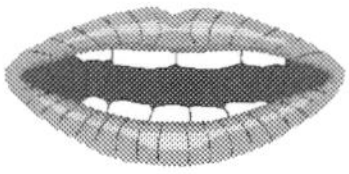

5.__________ 6.__________ 7.__________ 8.__________

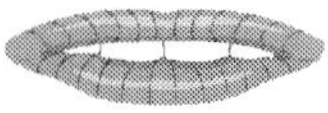
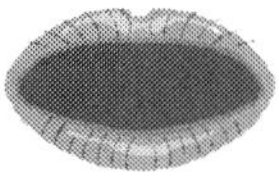
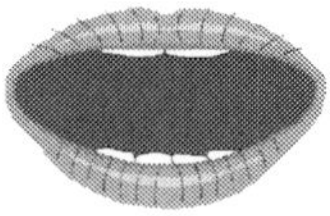
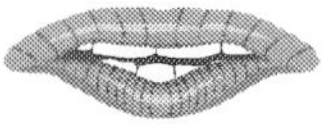

9.__________ 10.__________

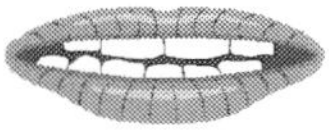
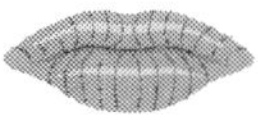

Solution:

8. plants

puzzle

The written list was:

Anthers, inner leaf, shoot, leaf, petal, ovary, root, stem, flower, wilting.

The words can be matched to their respective initial lip-shapes in the following order.

1. petal

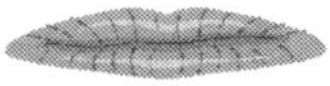

2. leaf

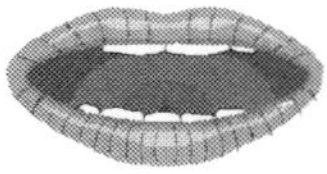

3. root

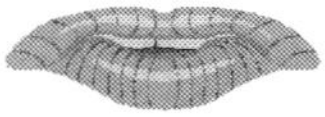

4. inner leaf

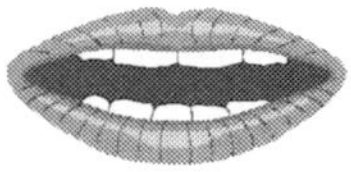

5. flower

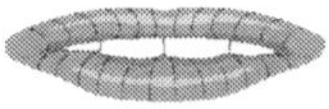

6. ovary

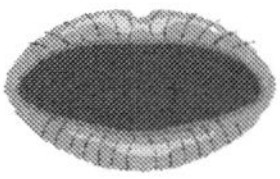

7. anthers

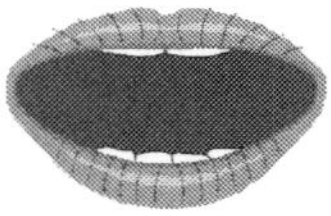

8. shoot

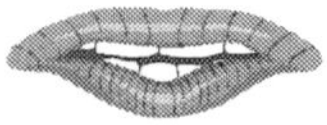

9. stem

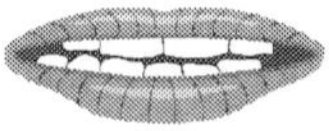

10. wilting

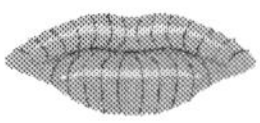

Lip-reading puzzle:

9. savings

The pictures below represent words to do with **savings** as a spoken list. The lip shape shown for each word is the first lip shape that would be seen by a lip-reader as the word is spoken.

Here are the words as a written list:
Annuity, interest, cheque, loan, money, overdraft, return, dividend, value, withdraw, yield.

Can you match the words on the list to the correct lip-shapes?

1.__________

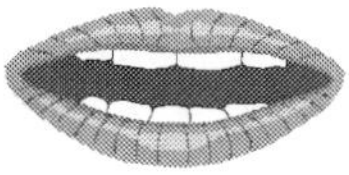

2.__________

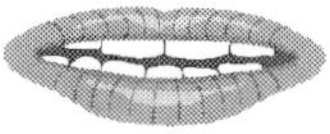

3.__________

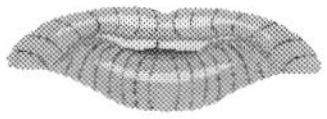

4.__________

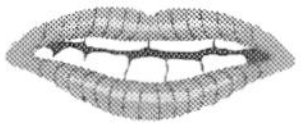

5.__________

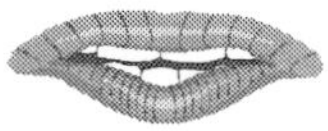

6.__________

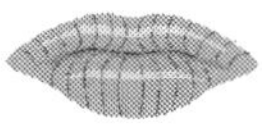

7.__________

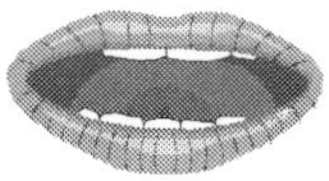

8.__________

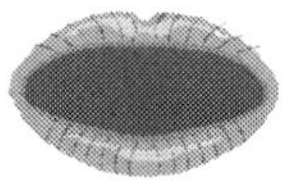

9.__________

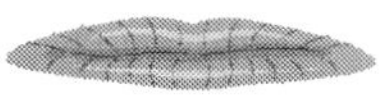

10.__________

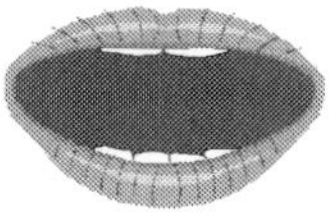

11.__________

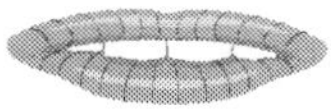

Solution:

9. savings

puzzle

The written list was:

Annuity, interest, cheque, loan, money, overdraft, return, dividend, value, withdraw, yield.

The words can be matched to their respective initial lip-shapes in the following order.

1.
interest

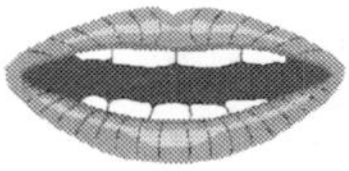

2.
dividend

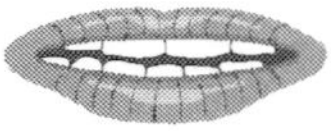

3.
return

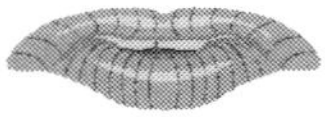

4.
yield

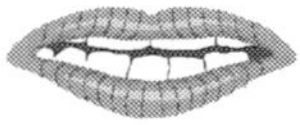

5.
cheque

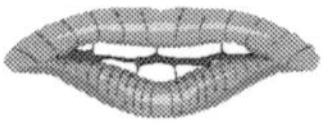

6.
withdraw

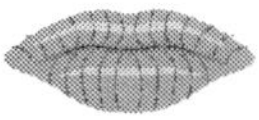

7.
loan

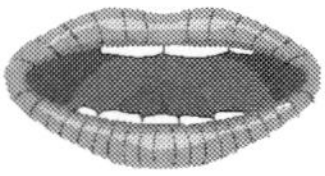

8.
overdraft

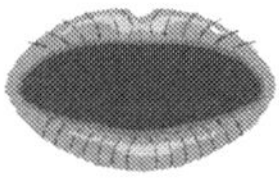

9.
money

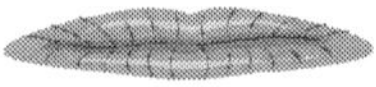

10.
annuity

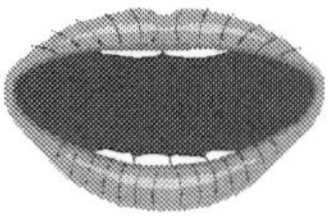

11.
value

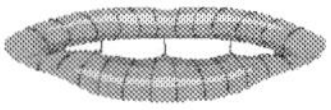

12.

Lip-reading puzzle:

10. sports

The pictures below represent names of **sports** as a spoken list. The lip shape shown for each word is the first that would be seen by a lip-reader.

Here are the words as a written list:
American football, water polo, long jump, shooting, basketball, rowing, off-piste skiing, tennis, volleyball.

Can you match the words on the list to the correct lip-shapes?

1.__________

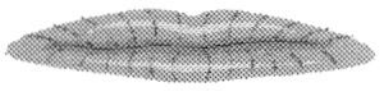

2.__________

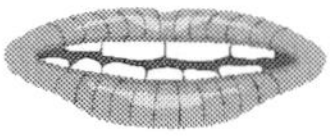

3.__________

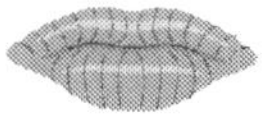

4.__________

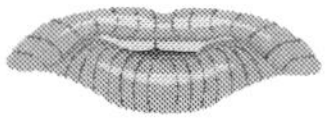

5.__________

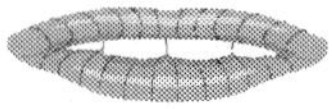

6.__________

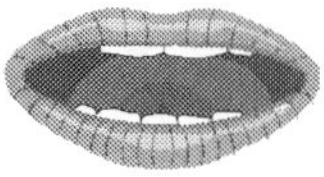

7.__________

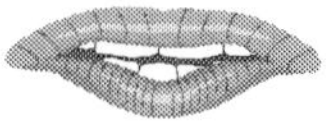

8.__________

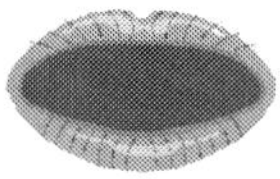

9.__________

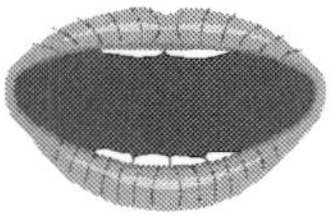

Solution:

10. sports

puzzle

The written list was:

American football, water polo, long jump, shooting, basketball, rowing, off-piste skiing, tennis, volleyball.

The words can be matched to their respective initial lip-shapes in the following order.

1.
basketball

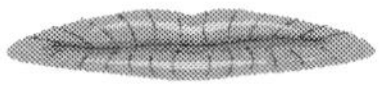

2.
tennis

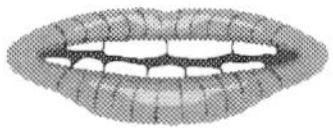

3.
water polo

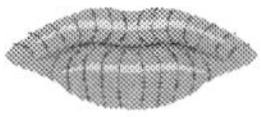

4.
rowing

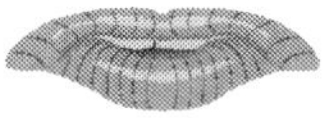

5.
volleyball

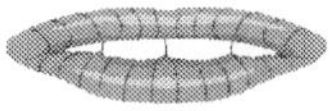

6.
long jump

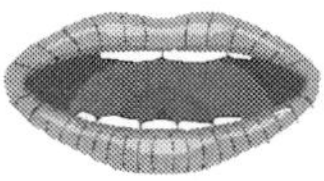

7.
shooting

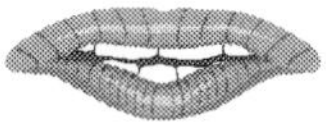

8.
off-piste skiing

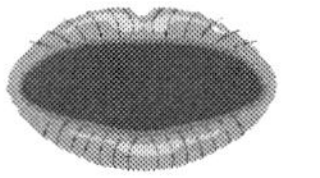

9.
American football

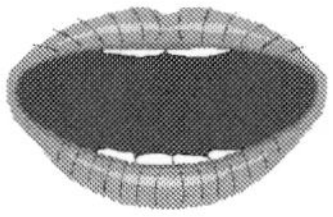

Lip-reading puzzle:

11. airports

The pictures below represent words used at **airports** as a spoken list. The lip shape shown for each word is the first lip shape that would be seen by a lip-reader as the word is spoken.

Here are the words as a written list:
Air crew, interchange, check-in, hostess, lounge, passport, security, duty free, transfer, flight.

Can you match the words on the list to the correct lip-shapes?

1.__________

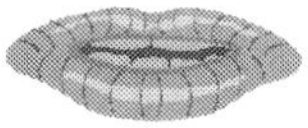

2.__________

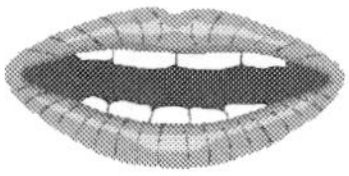

3.__________

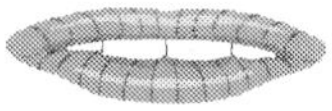

4.__________

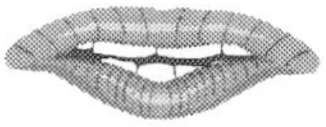

5.__________

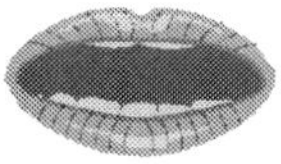

6.__________

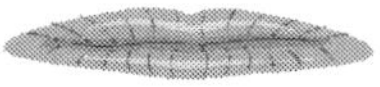

7.__________

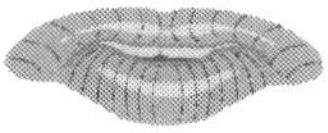

8.__________

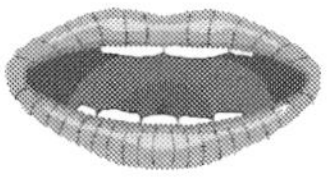

9.__________

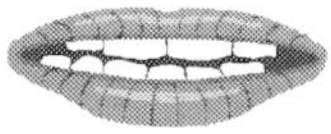

10.__________

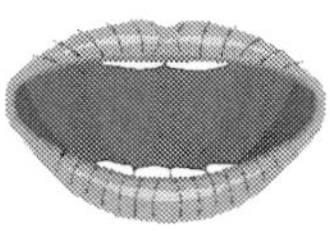

Solution:

11. airports

puzzle

The written list was:

Air crew, interchange, check-in, hostess, lounge, passport, security, duty free, transfer, flight.

The words can be matched to their respective initial lip-shapes in the following order.

1. duty free

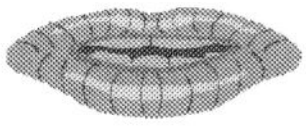

2. interchange

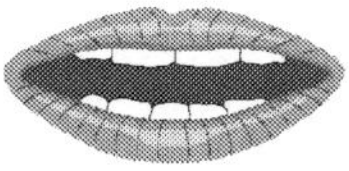

3. flight

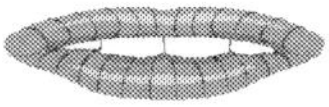

4. check-in

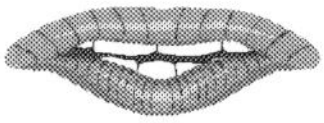

5. hostess

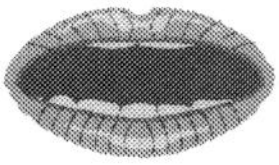

6. passport

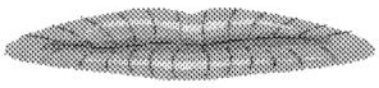

7. transfer

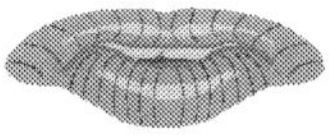

8. lounge

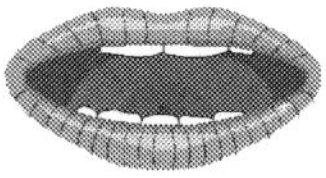

9. security

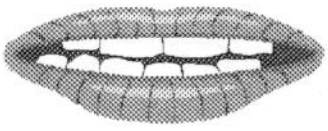

10. air crew

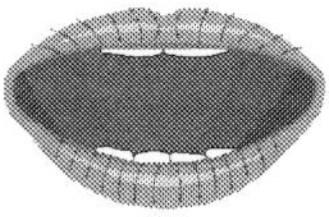

Lip-reading puzzle:

12. bumblebees

The pictures below represent words to do with **bumblebees** as a spoken list. The lip shape shown for each word is the first lip shape that would be seen by a lip-reader as the word is spoken.

The words are:

All brown, buff tailed, chestnut, clover, dandelion, lavender, orange tailed, rose, thistle, veronica, white tailed, yarrow.

Can you match the words on the list to the correct lip-shapes?

1.__________ 2.__________ 3.__________ 4.__________

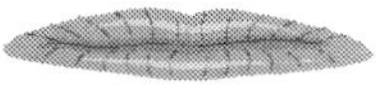
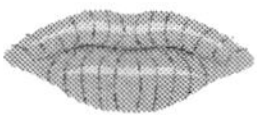
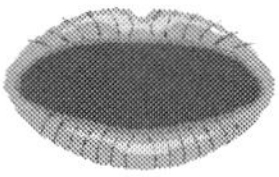
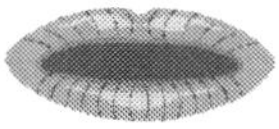

5.__________ 6.__________ 7.__________ 8.__________

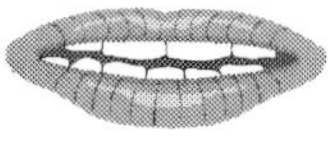
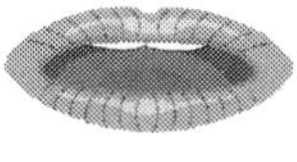
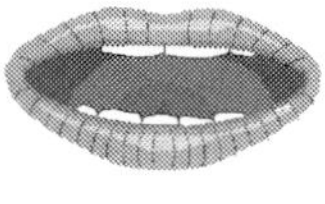
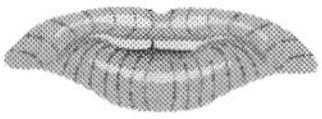

9.__________ 10.__________ 11.__________ 12.__________

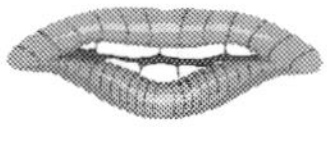
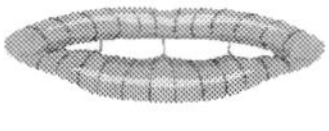
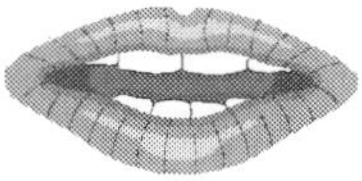
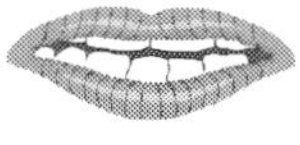

Solution:

12. bumblebees

puzzle

The written list was:

All brown, buff tailed, chestnut, clover, dandelion, lavender, orange tailed, rose, thistle, veronica, white tailed, yarrow.

The words can be matched to their respective initial lip-shapes in the following order.

1.
buff tailed

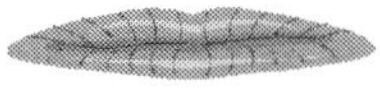

2.
white tailed

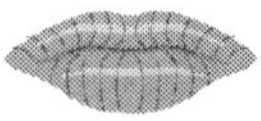

3.
orange tailed

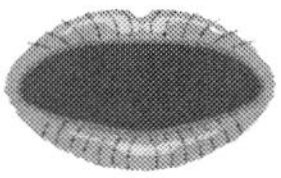

4.
all brown

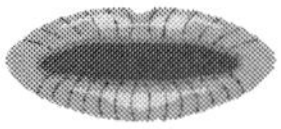

5.
dandelion

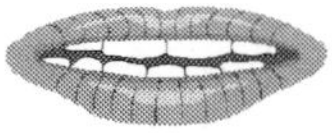

6.
clover

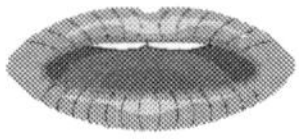

7.
lavender

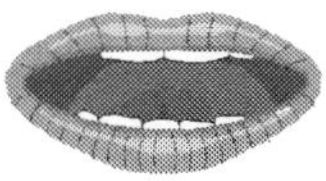

8.
rose

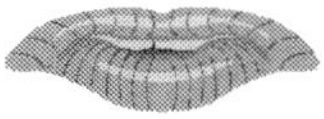

9.
chestnut

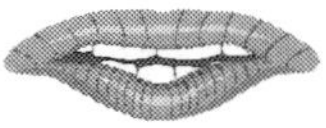

10.
veronica

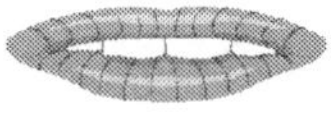

11.
thistle

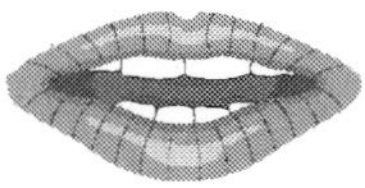

12.
yarrow

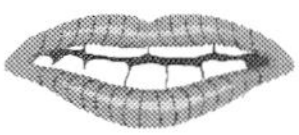

Lip-reading puzzle:

13. cakes

The pictures below represent words describing types of **cakes** as a spoken list. The lip shape shown for each word is the first a lip-reader would see.

Here are the words as a written list:
Jam sponge, gateau, Christmas cake, cup cake, layer cake, Battenburg, fairy cake, wedding cake, rich fruit cake, stollen.

Can you match the words on the list to the correct lip-shapes?

1.__________ 2.__________ 3.__________ 4.__________

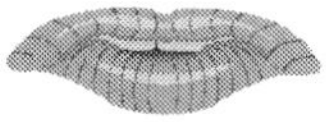
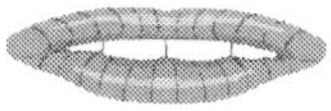
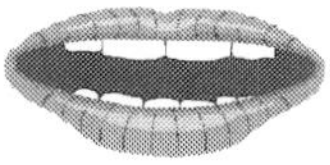
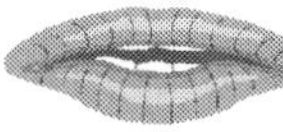

5.__________ 6.__________ 7.__________ 8.__________

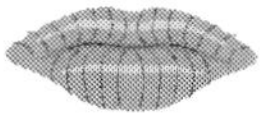
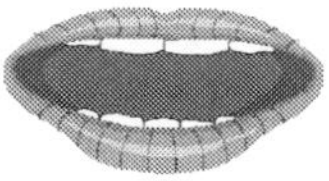
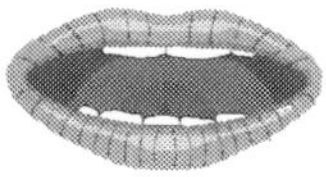

9.__________ 10.__________

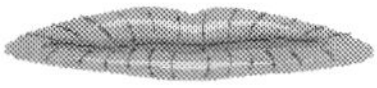
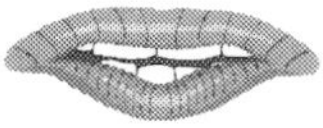

Solution:

13. cakes

puzzle

The written list was:

Jam sponge, gateau, Christmas cake, cup cake, layer cake, Battenburg, fairy cake, wedding cake, rich fruit cake, stollen.

The words can be matched to their respective initial lip-shapes in the following order.

1.
rich fruit cake

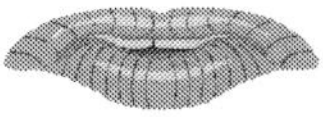

2.
fairy cake

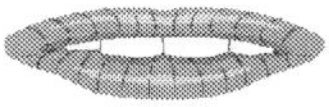

3.
gateau

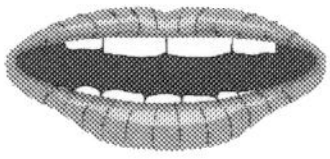

4.
Christmas cake

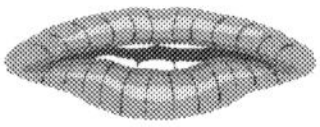

5.
wedding cake

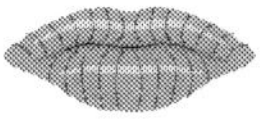

6.
stollen

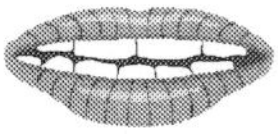

7.
cup cake

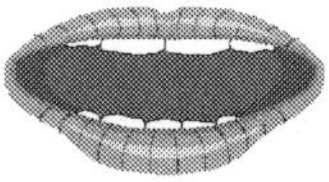

8.
layer cake

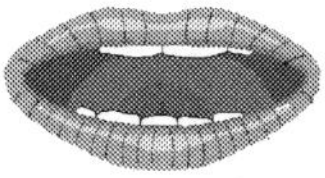

9.
Battenburg

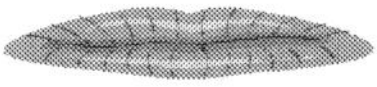

10.
Jam sponge

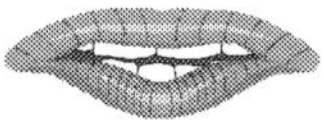

Lip-reading puzzle:

14. capital cities

The pictures below represent names of **capital cities** as a spoken list. The lip shape shown for each is the first lip shape that would be seen by a lip-reader when the name is spoken.

Here are the words as a written list:
Athens, Canberra, Gibraltar, Winnipeg, Lisbon, Berlin, Rome, Dublin, Freetown, Warsaw.

Can you match the words on the list to the correct lip-shapes?

1.__________ 2.__________ 3.__________ 4.__________

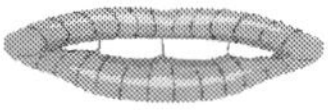
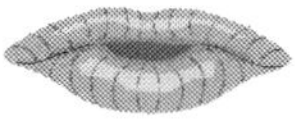
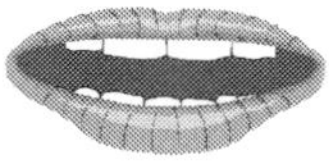
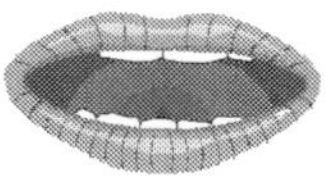

5.__________ 6.__________ 7.__________ 8.__________

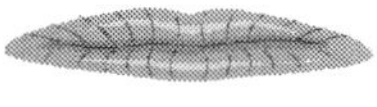
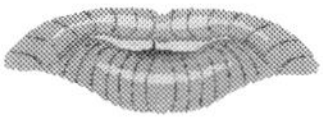
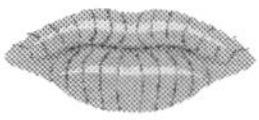
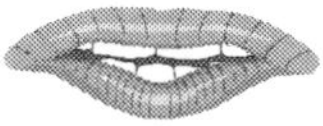

9.__________ 10.__________

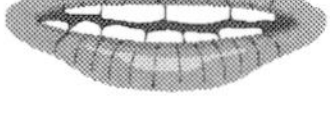
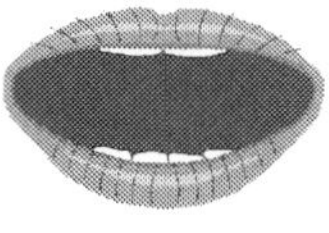

Solution:

14. *capital cities*

puzzle

The written list was:

Athens, Canberra, Gibraltar, Winnipeg, Lisbon, Berlin, Rome, Dublin, Freetown, Warsaw.

The words can be matched to their respective initial lip-shapes in the following order.

1.
Freetown

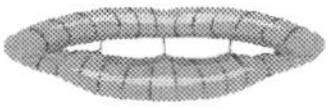

2.
Warsaw

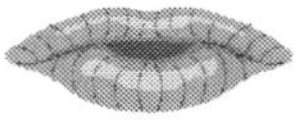

3.
Canberra

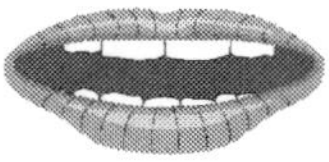

4.
Lisbon

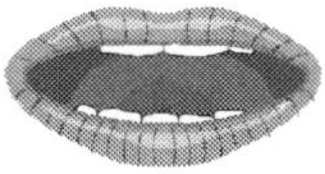

5.
Berlin

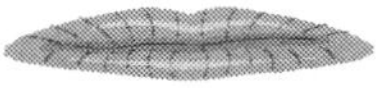

6.
Rome

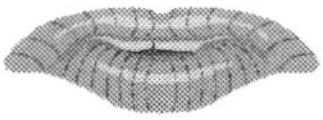

7.
Winnipeg

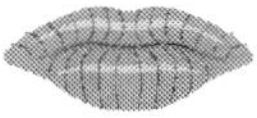

8.
Gibraltar

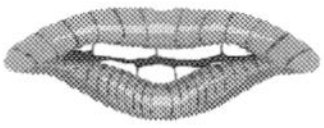

9.
Dublin

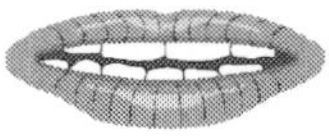

10.
Athens

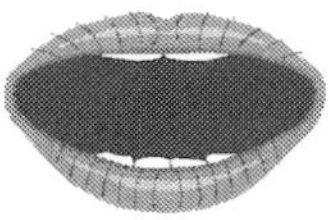

Lip-reading puzzle:

15. car parking

The pictures below represent words to do with **car parking** as a spoken list. The lip shape shown for each word is the first lip shape that would be seen by a lip-reader as the word is spoken.

Here are the words as a written list:

Off-street, warden, ticket, multi-storey, fines, arrival time, yellow lines, regulations, lost keys, charges.

Can you match the words on the list to the correct lip-shapes?

1.__________ 2.__________ 3.__________ 4.__________

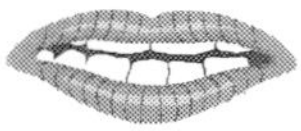
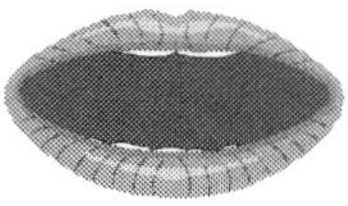
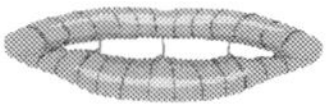
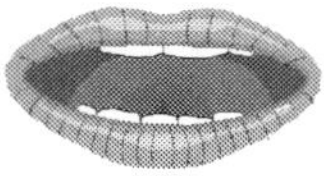

5.__________ 6.__________ 7.__________ 8.__________

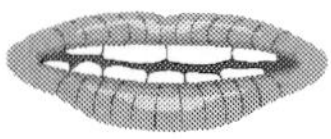
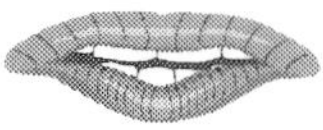
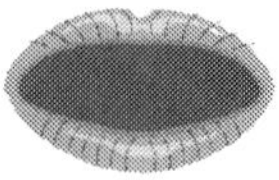

9.__________ 10.__________

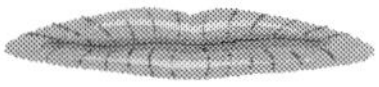
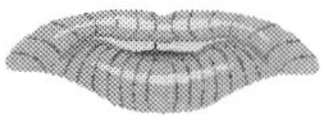

Solution:

15. car parking

puzzle

The written list was:

Off-street, warden, ticket, multi-storey, fines, arrival time, yellow lines, regulations, lost keys, charges.

The words can be matched to their respective initial lip-shapes in the following order.

1. yellow lines

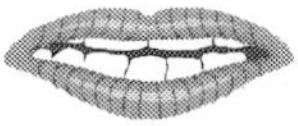

2. arrival time

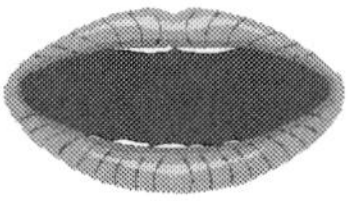

3. fines

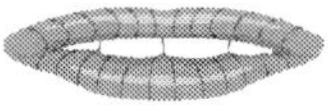

4. lost keys

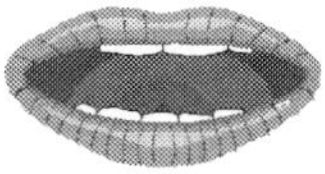

5. warden

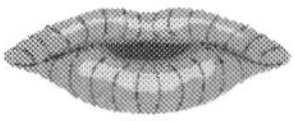

6. ticket

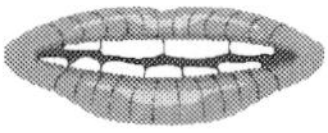

7. charges

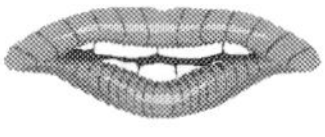

8. off-street

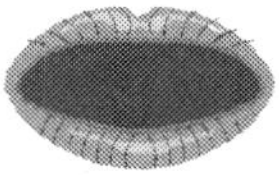

9. multi-storey

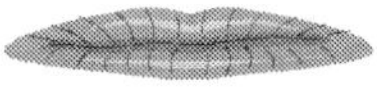

10. regulations

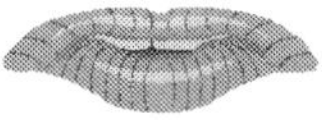

Lip-reading puzzle:

16. car servicing

The pictures below represent words that are used in **car servicing** as a spoken list. The lip shape shown for each word is the first lip shape that would be seen by a lip-reader as the word is spoken.

Here are the words as a written list:
Brake pads, clutch, computer, emissions, fuel cap, ignition, jack, lock, terminal, wipers, wrench.

Can you match the words on the list to the correct lip-shapes?

1.__________ 2.__________ 3.__________ 4.__________

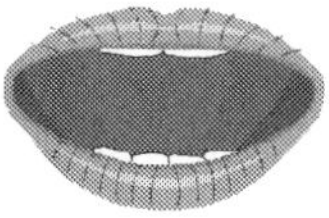
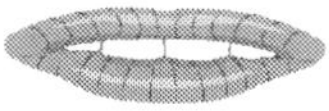
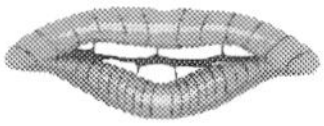
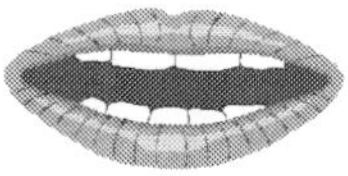

5.__________ 6.__________ 7.__________ 8.__________

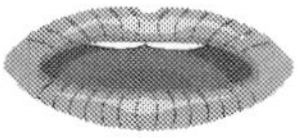
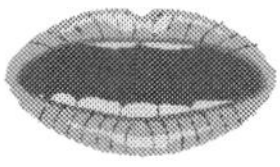
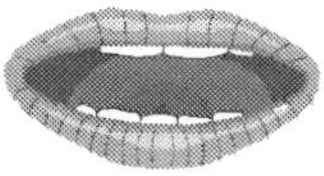
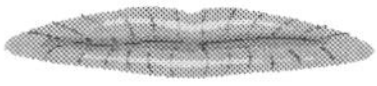

9.__________ 10.__________ 11.__________

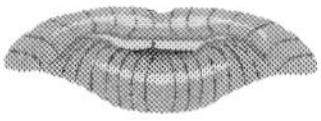
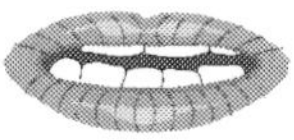
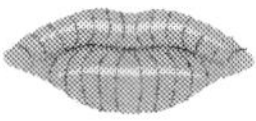

Solution:

16. car servicing

puzzle

The written list was:

Brake pads, clutch, computer, emissions, fuel cap, ignition, jack, lock, terminal, wipers, wrench.

The words can be matched to their respective initial lip-shapes in the following order.

1. emissions

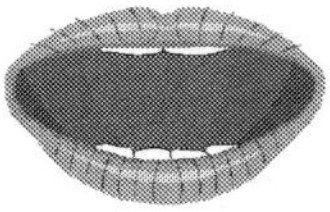

2. fuel cap

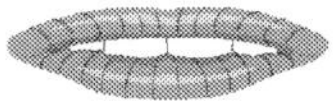

3. jack

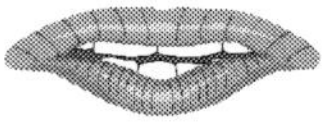

4. ignition

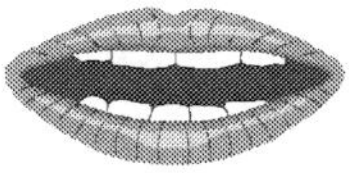

5. clutch

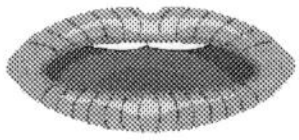

6. computer

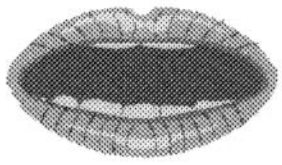

7. lock

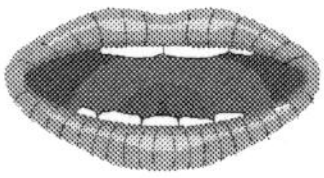

8. brake-pads

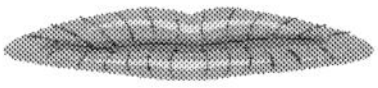

9. wrench

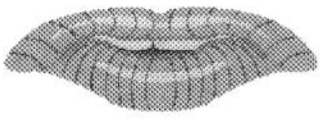

10. terminal

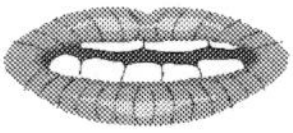

11. wipers

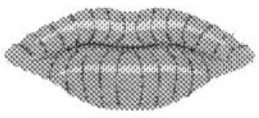

Lip-reading puzzle:

17. college study

The pictures below represent words to do with **college study** as a spoken list. The lip shape shown for each is the first seen by a lip-reader.

Here are the words as a written list:
Application, calculation, college, interview, choice, university, lecture, books, revision, study, examinations.

Can you match the words on the list to the correct lip-shapes?

1.__________ 2.__________ 3.__________ 4.__________

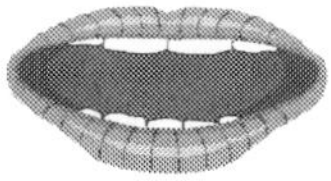
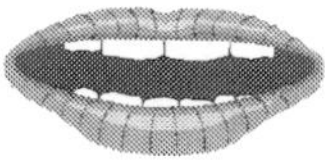
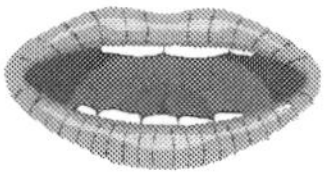
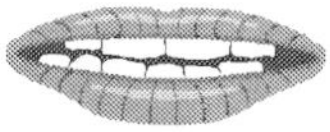

5.__________ 6.__________ 7.__________ 8.__________

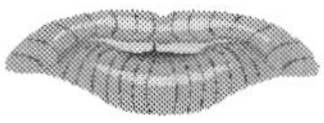
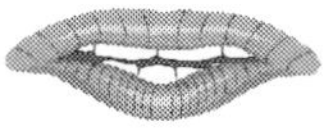
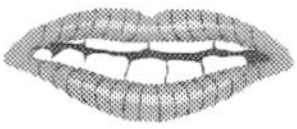
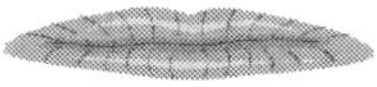

9.__________ 10.__________ 11.__________

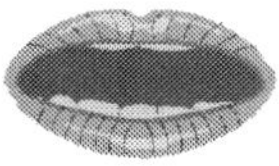
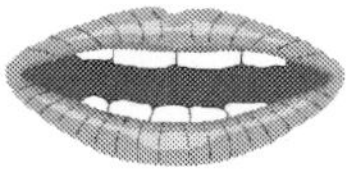
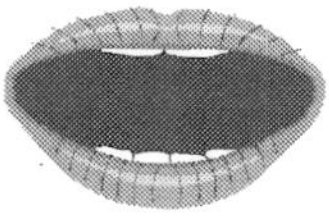

Solution:

17. college study

puzzle

The written list was:

Application, calculation, college, interview, choice, university, lecture, books, revision, study, examinations.

The words can be matched to their respective initial lip-shapes in the following order.

1. examinations

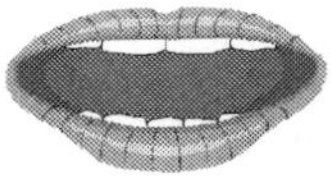

2. calculation

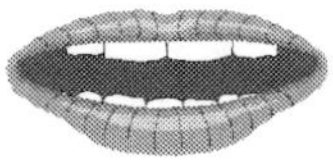

3. lecture

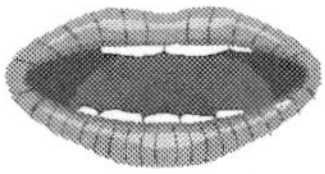

4. study

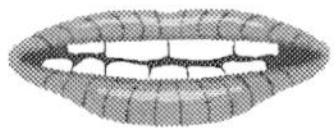

5. revision

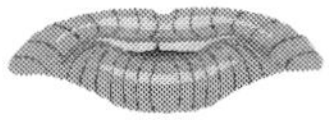

6. choice

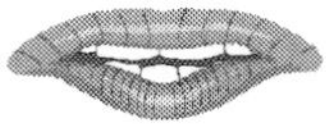

7. university

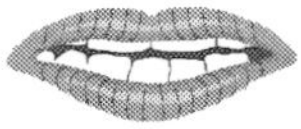

8. books

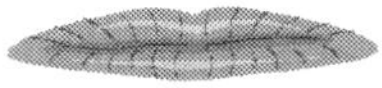

9. college

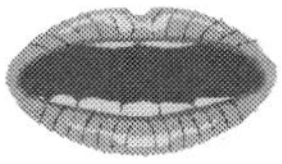

10. interview

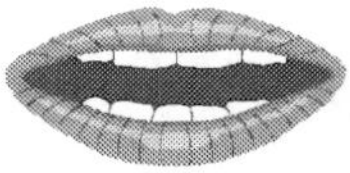

11. application

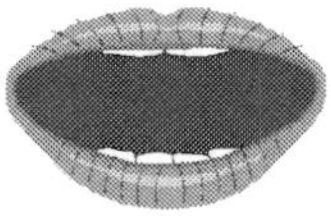

Lip-reading puzzle:

18. colours

The pictures below represent names of **colours** as a spoken list. The lip shape shown for each colour is the first that would be seen by a lip-reader when the word is spoken.

Here are the words as a written list:
Amber, cherry, gold, green, lime, magenta, orange, red, cyan, fuchsia, white, yellow.

Can you match the words on the list to the correct lip-shapes?

1.__________ 2.__________ 3.__________ 4.__________

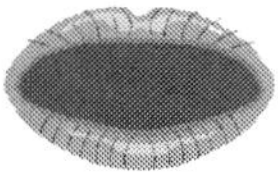
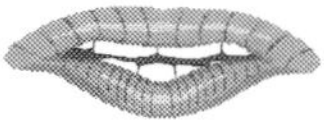
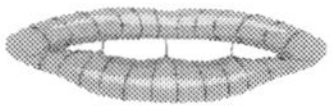
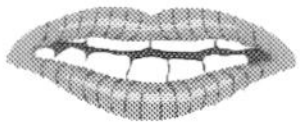

5.__________ 6.__________ 7.__________ 8.__________

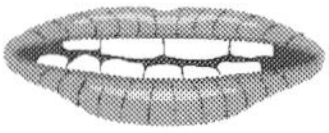
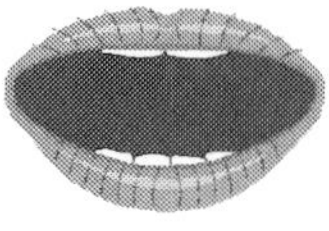
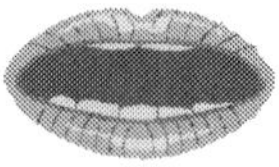
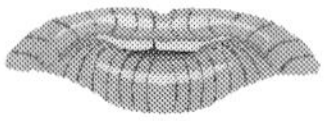

9.__________ 10.__________ 11.__________ 12__________

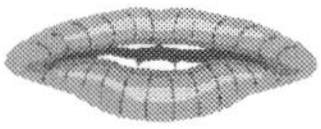
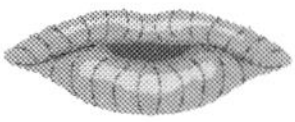
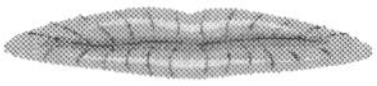
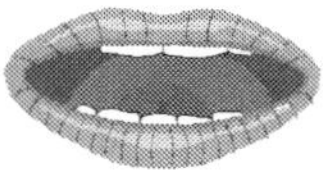

Solution:

18. colours

puzzle

The written list was:

Amber, cherry, gold, green, lime, magenta, orange, red, cyan, fuchsia, white, yellow.

The words can be matched to their respective initial lip-shapes in the following order.

1\. orange

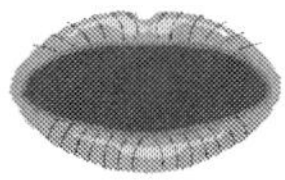

2\. cherry

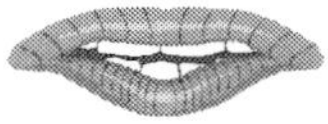

3\. fuchsia

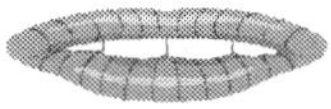

4\. yellow

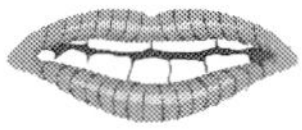

5\. cyan

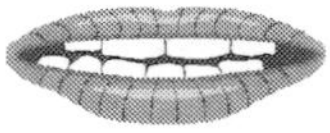

6\. amber

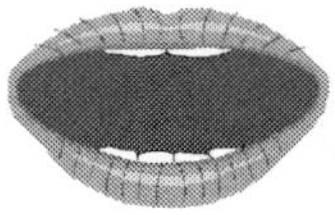

7\. gold

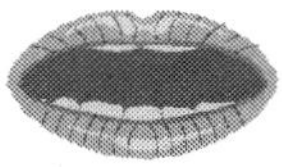

8\. red

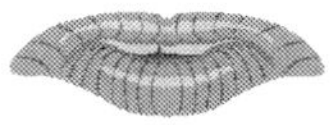

9\. green

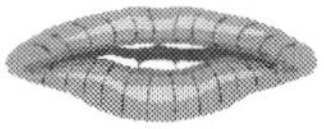

10\. white

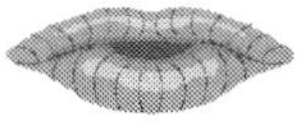

11\. magenta

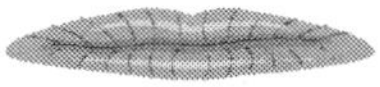

12\. lime

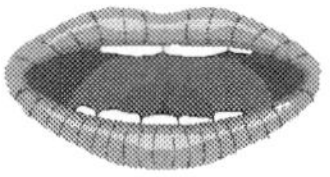

Lip-reading puzzle:

19. dog breeds

The pictures below represent names of **dog breeds** as a spoken list. The lip shape shown for each name is the first one a lip-reader would see.

Here are the words as a written list:
Airedale Terrier, English Bulldog, Jack Russell, Boxer, Cairn Terrier, Collie, Greyhound, Labrador, Whippet, Rottweiler, Gordon Setter.

Can you match the words on the list to the correct lip-shapes?

1.__________ 2.__________ 3.__________ 4.__________

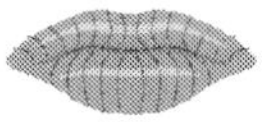
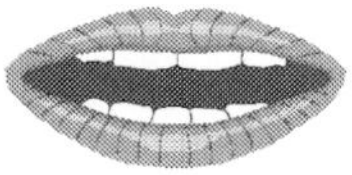
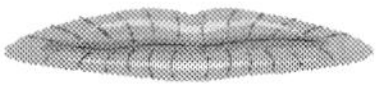
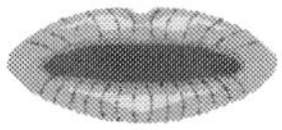

5.__________ 6.__________ 7.__________ 8.__________

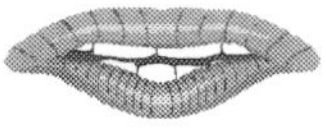
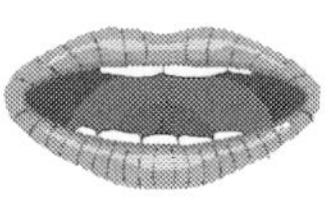
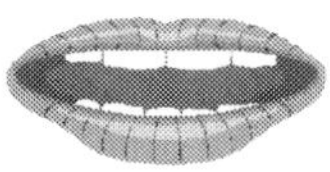
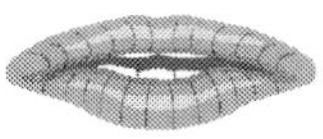

9.__________ 10.__________ 11.__________

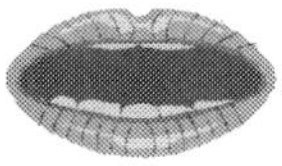
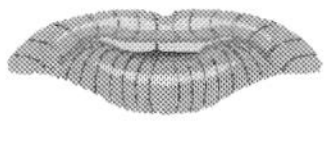
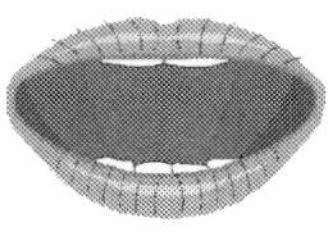

Solution:

19. dog breeds

puzzle

The written list was:

Airedale Terrier, English Bulldog, Jack Russell, Boxer, Cairn Terrier, Collie, Greyhound, Labrador, Whippet, Rottweiler, Gordon Setter.

The words can be matched to their respective initial lip-shapes in the following order.

1. Whippet

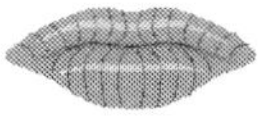

2. English Bulldog

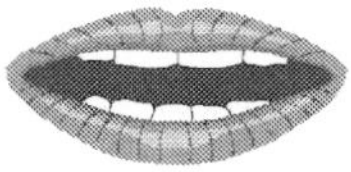

3. Boxer

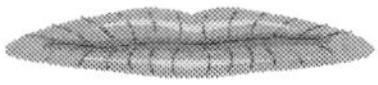

4. Gordon Setter

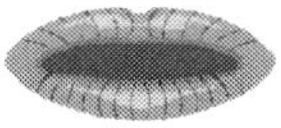

5. Jack Russell

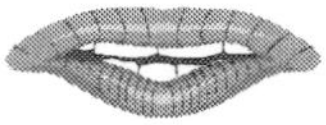

6. Labrador

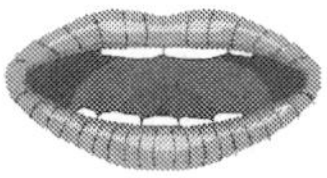

7. Cairn Terrier

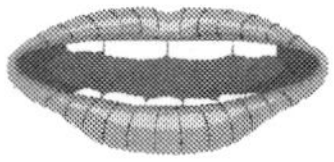

8. Greyhound

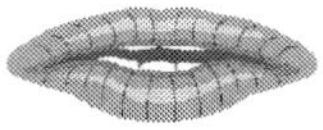

9. Collie

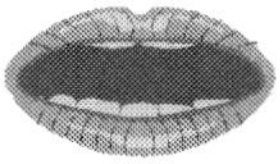

10. Rottweiler

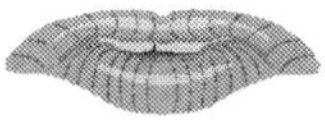

11. Airedale Terrier

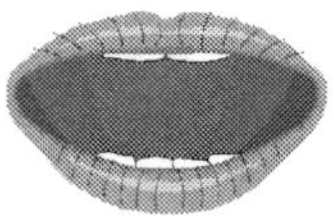

Lip-reading puzzle:

20. edible nuts

The pictures below represent words to do with **edible nuts** as a spoken list. The lip shape shown for each word is the first lip shape that would be seen by a lip-reader as the word is spoken.

Here are the words as a written list:
Almond, chestnut, Brazil nut, cob nut, walnut, filbert, cashew, groundnut, redskin peanut..

Can you match the words on the list to the correct lip-shapes?

1.__________

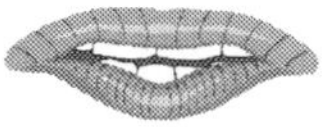

2.__________

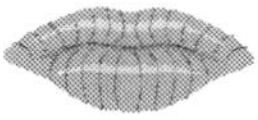

3.__________

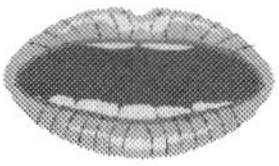

4.__________

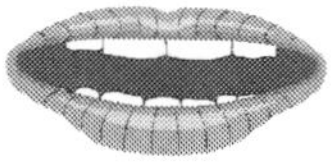

5.__________

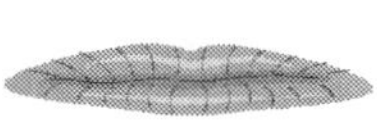

6.__________

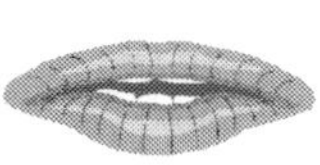

7.__________

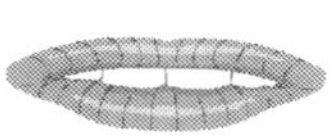

8.__________

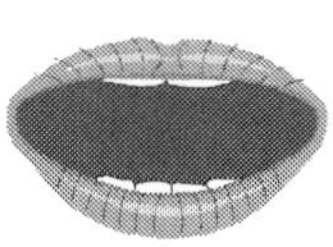

9.__________

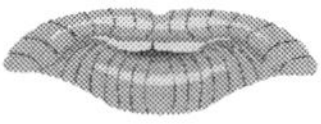

Solution:

20. edible nuts

puzzle

The written list was:

Almond, chestnut, Brazil nut, cob nut, walnut, filbert, cashew, groundnut, redskin peanut..

The words can be matched to their respective initial lip-shapes in the following order.

1.
chestnut

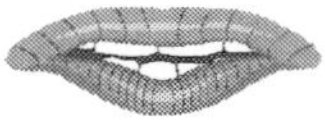

2.
walnut

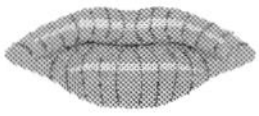

3.
cob nut

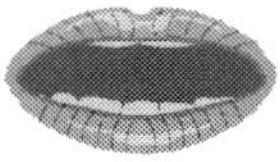

4.
cashew

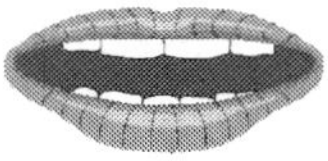

5.
Brazil nut

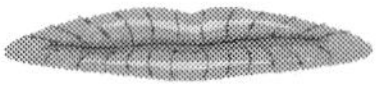

6.
ground nut

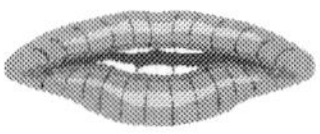

7.
filbert,

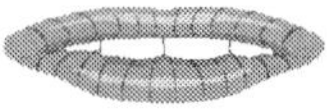

8.
almond

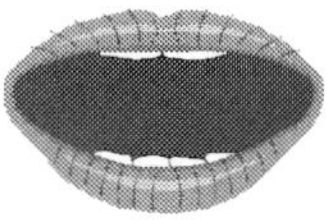

9.
redskin peanut

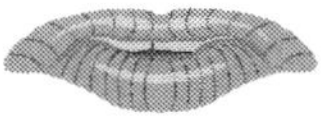

Lip-reading puzzle:

21. *fences*

The pictures below represent words describing types of **fences** as a spoken list. The lip shape shown for each word is the first the lip-reader sees.

Here are the words as a written list:
Acoustic, electric, chain-link, ha-ha, hedge, hurdle, close boarded, barbed wire, ring fence, stockade, wattle.

Can you match the words on the list to the correct lip-shapes?

1.__________ 2.__________ 3.__________ 4.__________

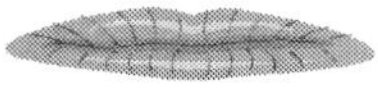
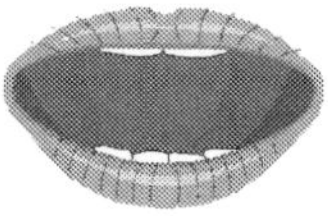
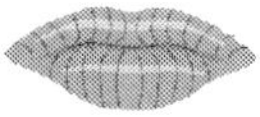
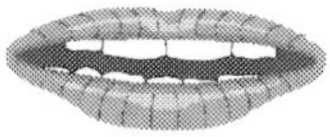

5.__________ 6.__________ 7.__________ 8.__________

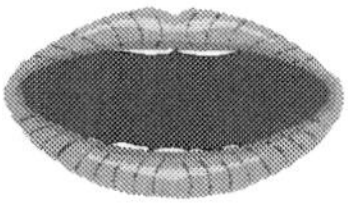
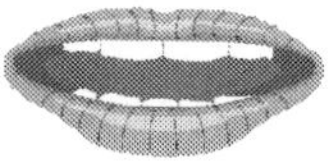
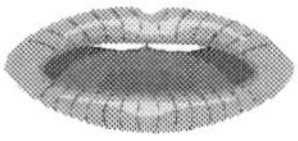
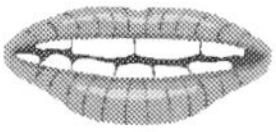

9.__________ 10.__________ 11.__________

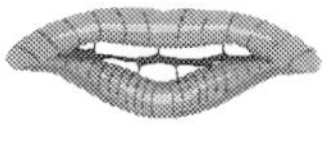
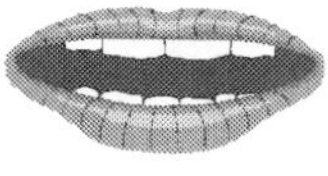
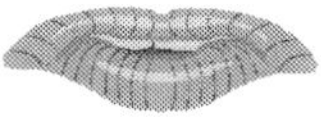

Solution:

21. fences

puzzle

The written list was:

Acoustic, electric, chain-link, ha-ha, hedge, hurdle, close boarded, barbed wire, ring fence, stockade, wattle.

The words can be matched to their respective initial lip-shapes in the following order.

1. barbed wire

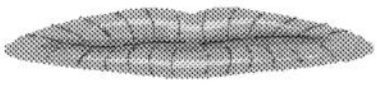

2. electric

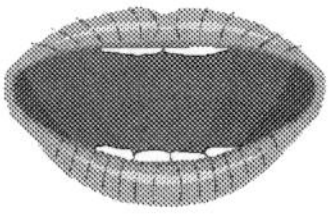

3. wattle

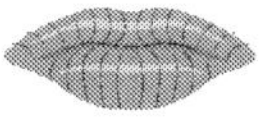

4. hurdle

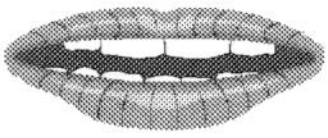

5. acoustic

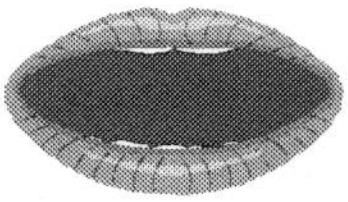

6. hedge

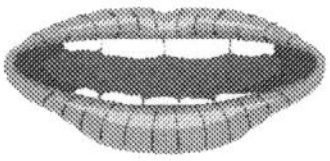

7. close boarded

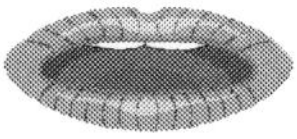

8. stockade

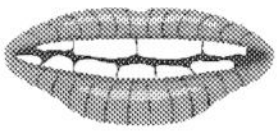

9. chain-link

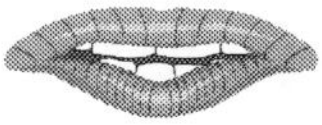

10. ha-ha

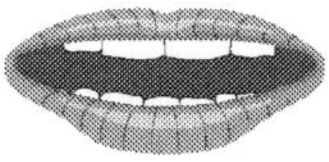

11. ring fence

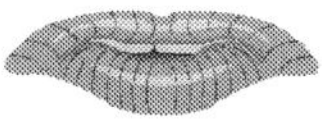

Lip-reading puzzle:

22. *fireworks*

The pictures below represent words to do with **fireworks** as a spoken list. The lip shape shown for each word is the first lip shape that would be seen by a lip-reader as the word is spoken.

Here are the words as a written list:
Jumping-jack, Catherine-wheel, lighter, mortar, rocket, squib, display, fountain, wheel, explosion

Can you match the words on the list to the correct lip-shapes?

1.__________ 2.__________ 3.__________ 4.__________

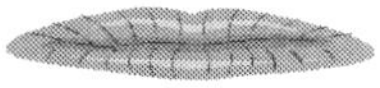
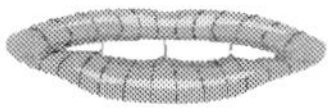
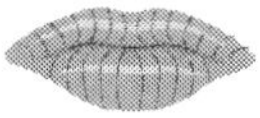
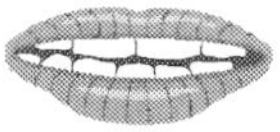

5.__________ 6.__________ 7.__________ 8.__________

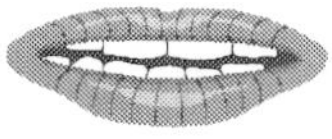
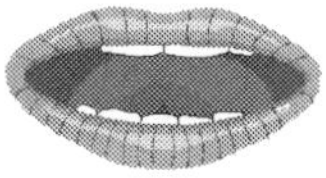
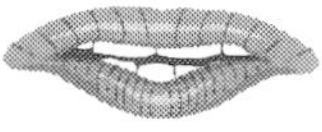
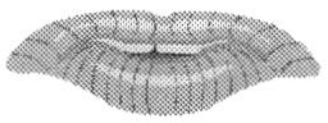

9.__________ 10.__________

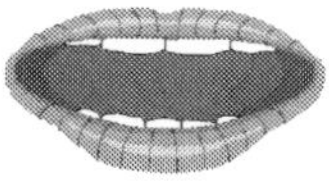
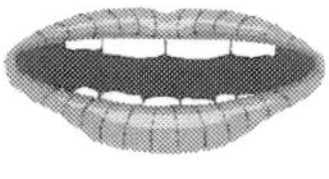

Solution:

22. fireworks

puzzle

The written list was:

Jumping-jack, Catherine-wheel, lighter, mortar, rocket, squib, display, fountain, wheel, explosion

The words can be matched to their respective initial lip-shapes in the following order.

1. mortar

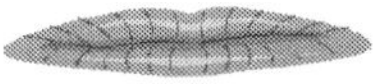

2. fountain

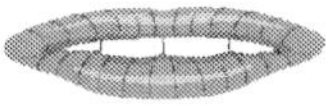

3. wheel

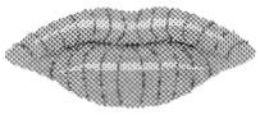

4. squib

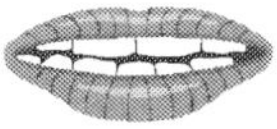

5. display

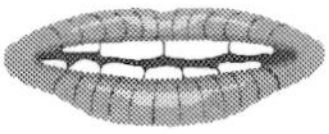

6. lighter

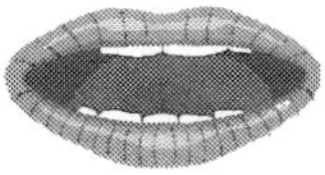

7. jumping-jack

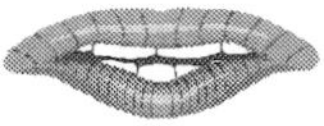

8. rocket

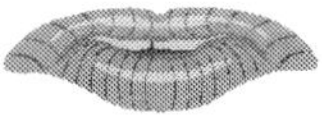

9. explosion

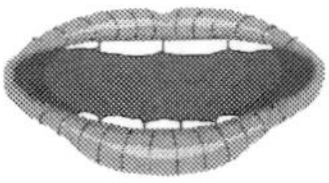

10. Catherine wheel

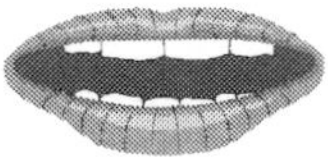

Lip-reading puzzle:

23. gardening

The pictures below represent words to do with **gardening** as a spoken list. The lip shape shown for each word is the first lip shape that would be seen by a lip-reader as the word is spoken.

Here are the words as a written list:
Hoe, spade, cloche, trowel, dock, germination, fertilizer, wheel-barrow, manure, greenhouse.

Can you match the words on the list to the correct lip-shapes?

1.__________ 2.__________ 3.__________ 4.__________

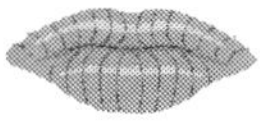 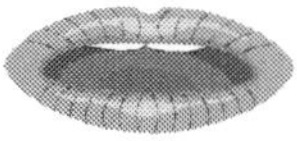 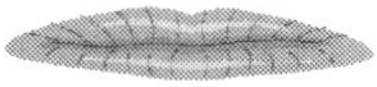 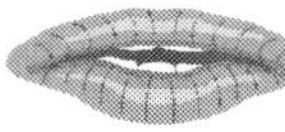

5.__________ 6.__________ 7.__________ 8.__________

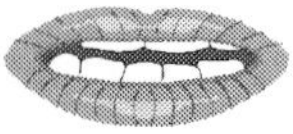 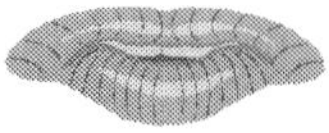 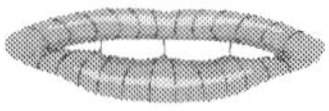 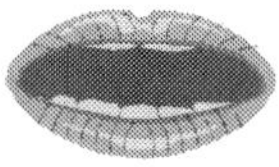

9.__________ 10.__________

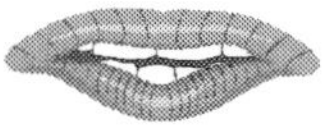 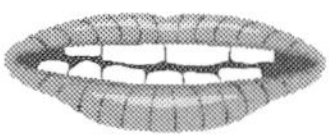

Solution:

23. gardening

puzzle

The written list was:

Hoe, spade, cloche, trowel, dock, germination, fertilizer, wheel-barrow, manure, greenhouse.

The words can be matched to their respective initial lip-shapes in the following order.

1. wheel-barrow

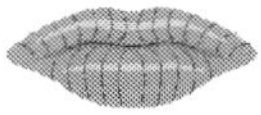

2. cloche

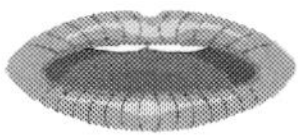

3. manure

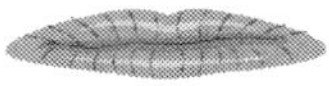

4. greenhouse

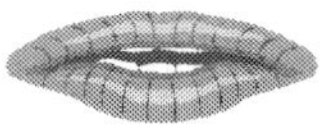

5. dock

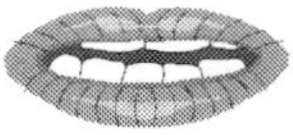

6. trowel

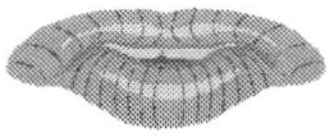

7. fertilizer

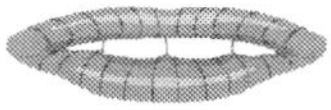

8. hoe

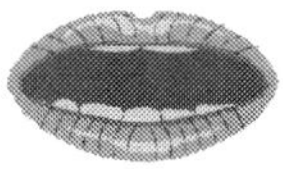

9. germination

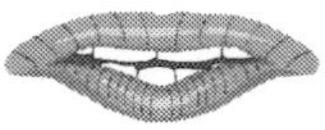

10. spade

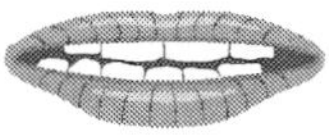

Lip-reading puzzle:

24. head-wear

The pictures below represent words describing types of **head-wear** as a spoken list. The lip shape shown is the first a lip-reader would see.

Here are the words as a written list:
Hard hat, cloche hat, racing helmet, cricket cap, Panama, turban, top hat, woollen hat, chef's hat, fez.

Can you match the words on the list to the correct lip-shapes?

1.__________ 2.__________ 3.__________ 4.__________

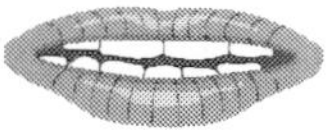
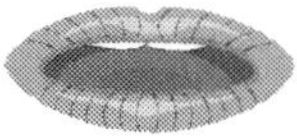
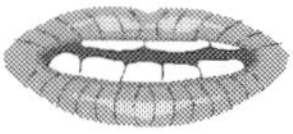
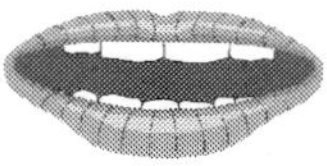

5.__________ 6.__________ 7.__________ 8.__________

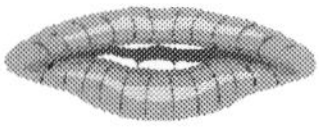
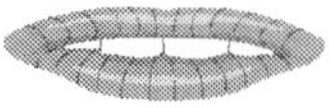
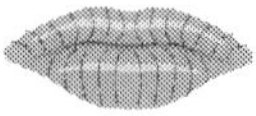
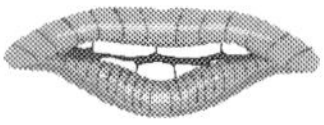

9.__________ 10.__________

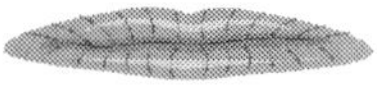
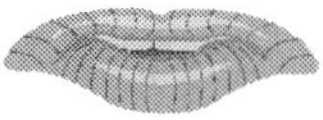

Solution:

24. head-wear

puzzle

The written list was:

Hard hat, cloche hat, racing helmet, cricket cap, Panama, turban, top hat, woollen hat, chef's hat, fez.

The words can be matched to their respective initial lip-shapes in the following order.

1. top hat

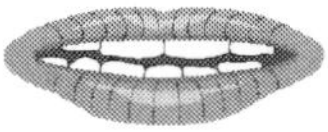

2. cloche hat

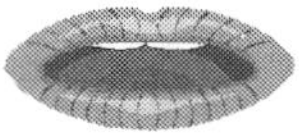

3. turban

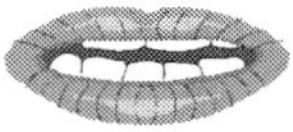

4. hard hat,

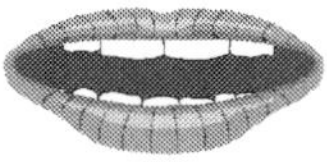

5. cricket cap

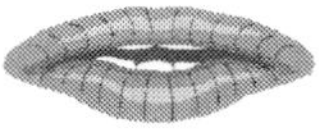

6. fez

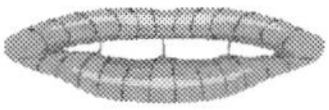

7. woollen hat

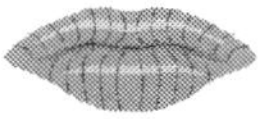

8. chef's hat

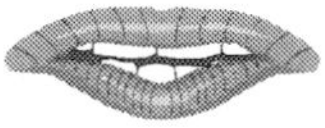

9. Panama

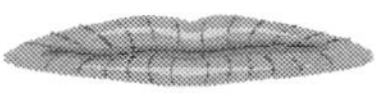

10. racing helmet

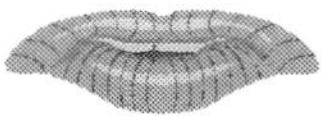

Lip-reading puzzle:

25. hiking

The pictures below represent words used when **hiking** as a spoken list. The lip shape shown is the first a lip-reader sees as the word is spoken.

Here are the words as a written list:
Compass, water course, gate, gradient, map, overgrown, rain-wear, shoreline, summit, unmarked, view-point.

Can you match the words on the list to the correct lip-shapes?

1.___________ 2.___________ 3.___________ 4.___________

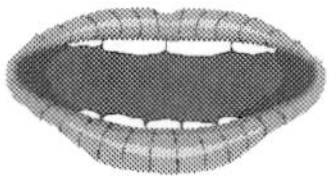
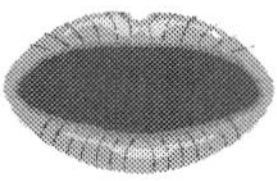
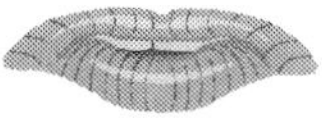
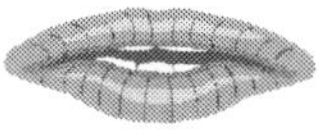

5.___________ 6.___________ 7.___________ 8.___________

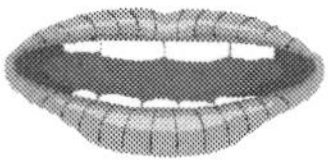
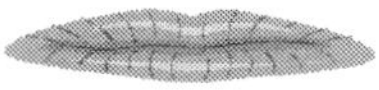
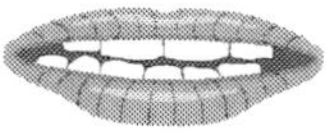
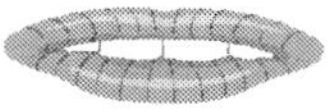

9.___________ 10.___________ 11.___________

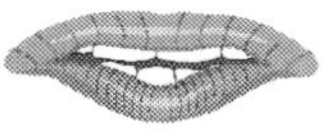
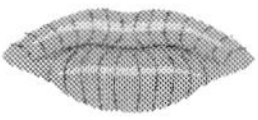
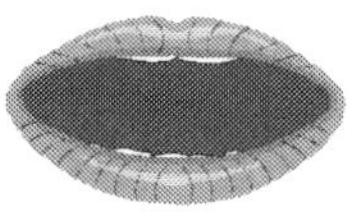

Solution:

25. hiking

puzzle

The written list was:

Compass, water course, gate, gradient, map, overgrown, rain-wear, shoreline, summit, unmarked, view-point,

The words can be matched to their respective initial lip-shapes in the following order.

1. compass

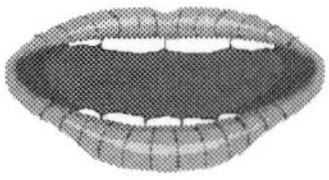

2. overgrown

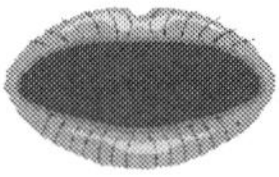

3. rain-wear

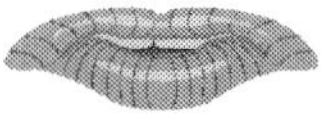

4. gradient

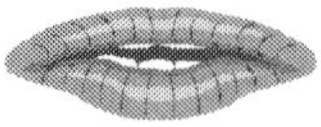

5. gate

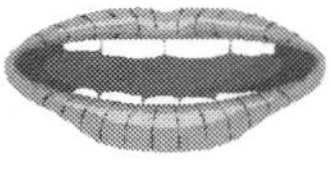

6. map

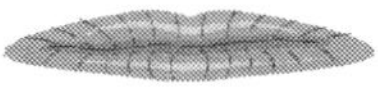

7. summit

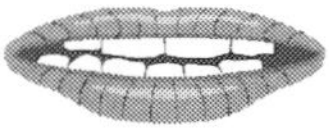

8. view-point

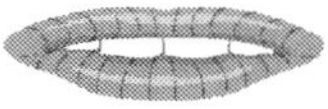

9. shoreline

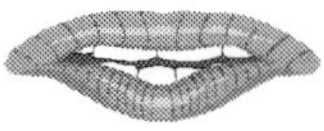

10. water course

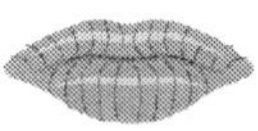

11. unmarked

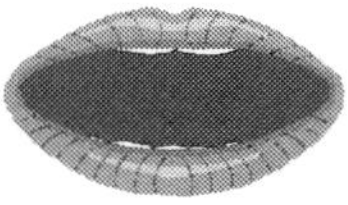

Lip-reading puzzle:

26. insects

The pictures below represent names of **insects** as a spoken list. The lip shape shown for each name is the first lip shape that would be seen by a lip-reader when it is spoken.

Here are the names as a written list:
Wasp, ant, earwig, house fly, grasshopper, hornet, locust, beetle, fly, dragonfly.

Can you match the names on the list to the correct lip-shapes?

1.__________ 2.__________ 3.__________ 4.__________

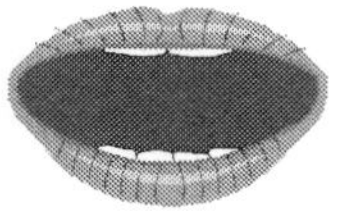
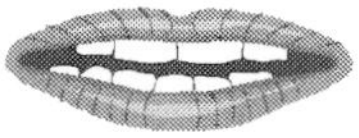
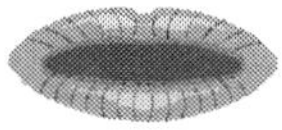
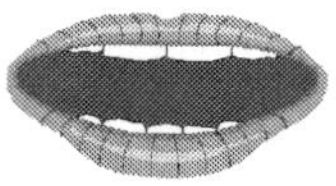

5.__________ 6.__________ 7.__________ 8.__________

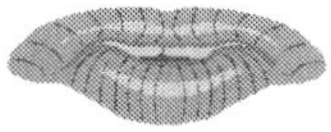
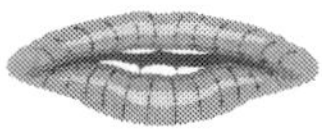
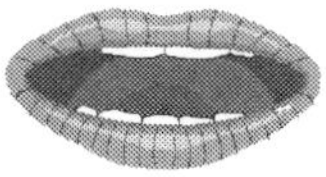
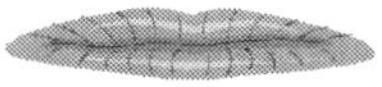

9.__________ 10.__________

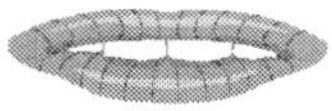
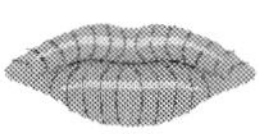

Solution:

26. insects

puzzle

The written list was:

Wasp, ant, earwig, house fly, grasshopper, hornet, locust, beetle, fly, dragonfly.

The names can be matched to their respective initial lip-shapes in the following order.

1.
ant

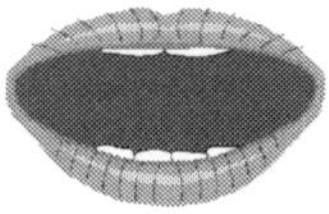

2.
earwig

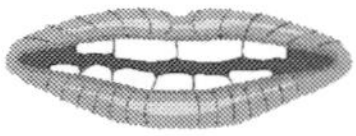

3.
hornet

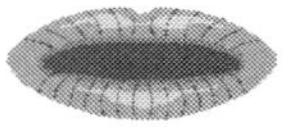

4.
house fly

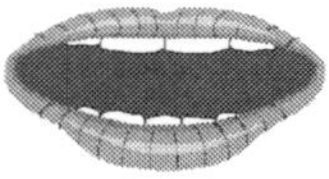

5.
dragonfly

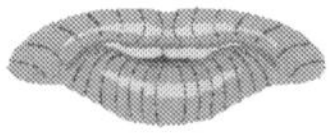

6.
grasshopper

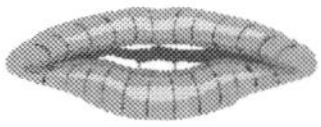

7.
locust

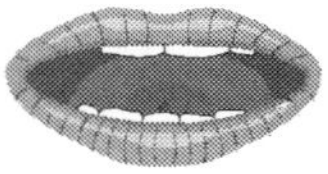

8.
beetle

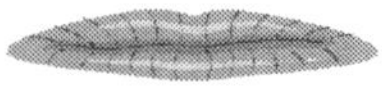

9.
fly

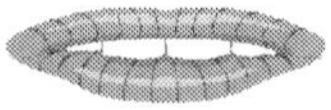

10.
wasp

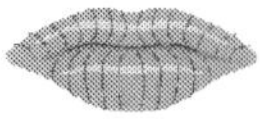

Lip-reading puzzle:

27. jewellery

The pictures below represent names of **jewellery** as a spoken list. The lip shape shown for each word is the first seen by a lip-reader as the word is spoken.

Here are the words as a written list:
Ring, bracelet, wedding ring, fáinne, necklace, lapel pin, cufflink, coronet, hairpin, shirt stud, anklet.

Can you match the words on the list to the correct lip-shapes?

1.__________ 2.__________ 3.__________ 4.__________

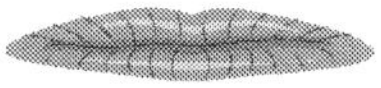
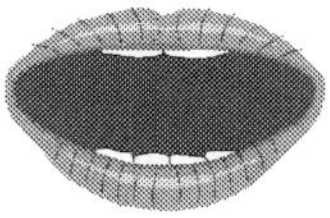
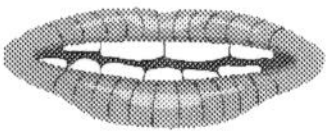
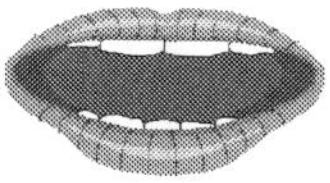

5.__________ 6.__________ 7.__________ 8.__________

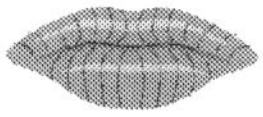
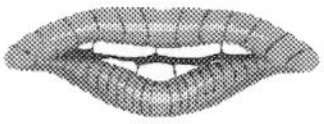
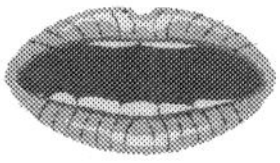
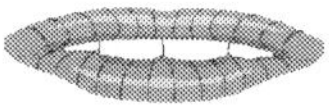

9.__________ 10.__________ 11.__________

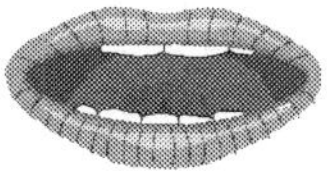
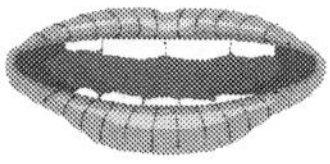
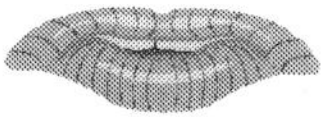

Solution:

27. jewellery

puzzle

The written list was:

Ring, bracelet, wedding ring, fáinne, necklace, lapel pin, cufflink, coronet, hairpin, shirt stud, anklet.

The words can be matched to their respective initial lip-shapes in the following order.

1.
bracelet

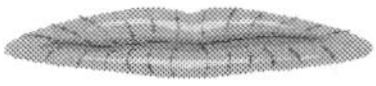

2.
anklet

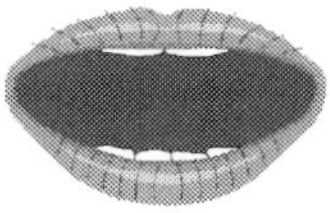

3.
necklace

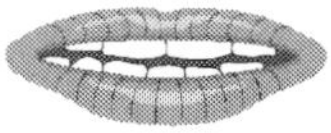

4.
cufflink

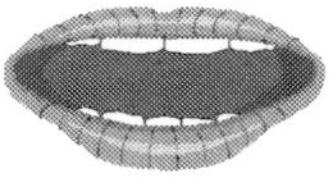

5.
wedding ring

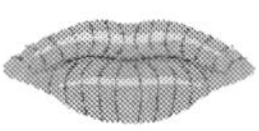

6.
shirt stud

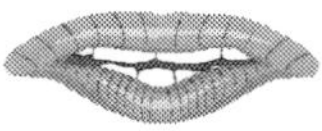

7.
coronet

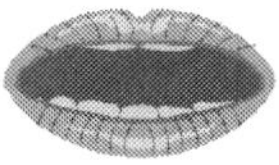

8.
fáinne

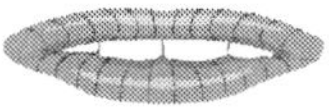

9.
lapel pin

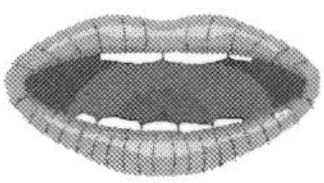

10.
hairpin

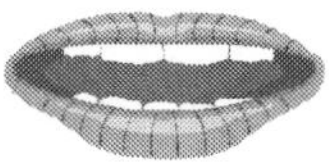

11.
ring

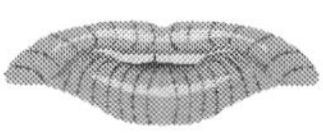

Lip-reading puzzle:

28. kitchen

The pictures below represent some names of **kitchen utensils** as a spoken list. The lip shape shown for each is the first seen by a lip-reader.

Here are the words as a written list:
Utensil, chopping board, hand whisk, colander, ladle, masher, rolling pin, spoon, thermometer, oven, fish scoop, whisk.

Can you match the words on the list to the correct lip-shapes?

1.__________ 2.__________ 3.__________ 4.__________

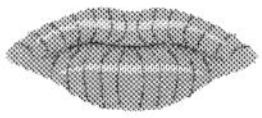
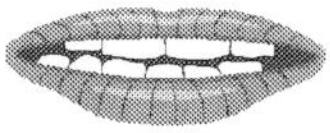
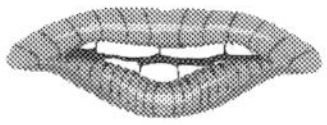
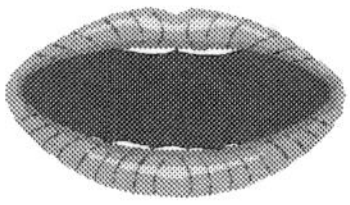

5.__________ 6.__________ 7.__________ 8.__________

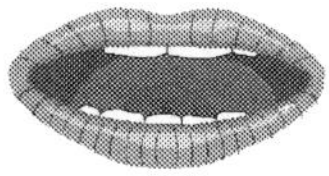
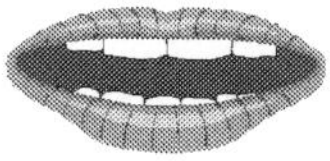
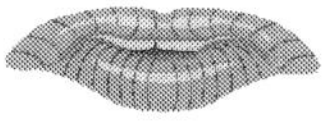
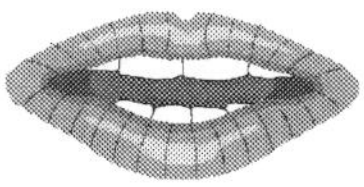

9.__________ 10.__________ 11.__________ 12.__________

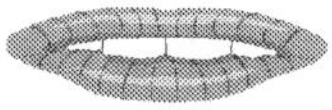
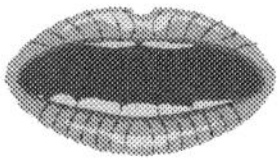
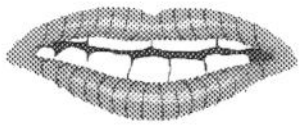
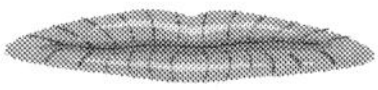

Solution:

28. kitchen

puzzle

The written list was:

Utensil, chopping board, hand whisk, colander, ladle, masher, rolling pin, spoon, thermometer, oven, fish scoop, whisk.

The words can be matched to their respective initial lip-shapes in the following order.

1. whisk

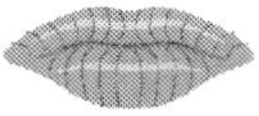

2. spoon

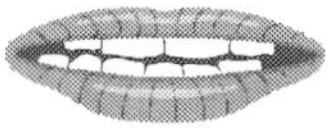

3. chopping board

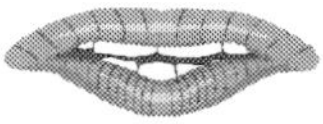

4. oven

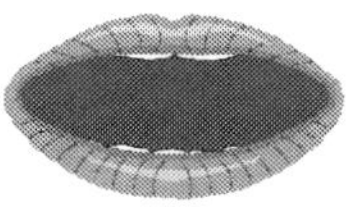

5. ladle

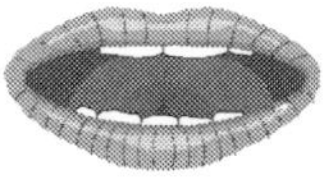

6. hand whisk

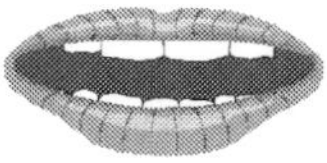

7. rolling pin

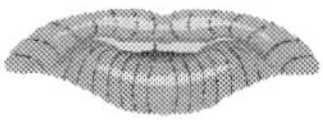

8. thermometer

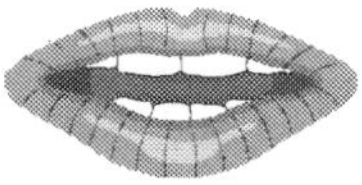

9. fish scoop

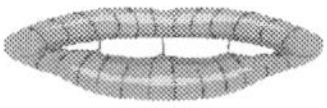

10. colander

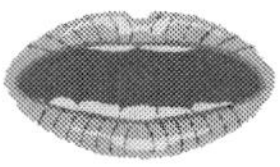

11. utensil

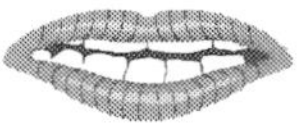

12. masher,

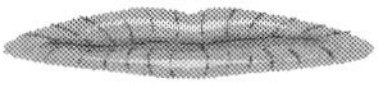

Lip-reading puzzle:

29. knitting

The pictures below represent words to do with **knitting** as a spoken list. The lip shape shown for each word is the first lip shape that would be seen by a lip-reader as the word is spoken.

Here are the words as a written list:
Cast-off, clustering, Fair-Isle, loops, pattern, ribbing, smocking, twist, welting, yarn.

Can you match the words on the list to the correct lip-shapes?

1.__________ 2.__________ 3.__________ 4.__________

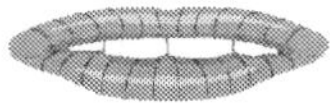 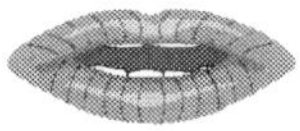 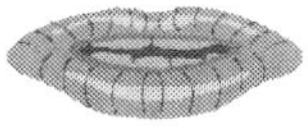 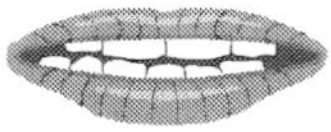

5.__________ 6.__________ 7.__________ 8.__________

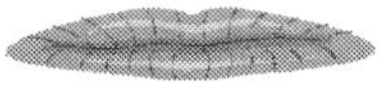 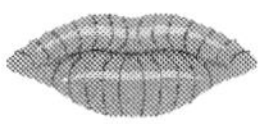 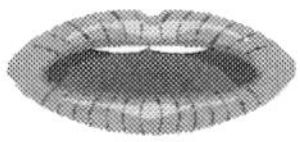 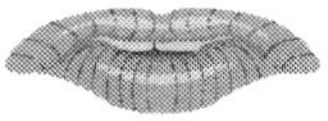

9.__________ 10.__________

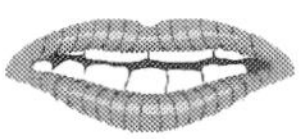 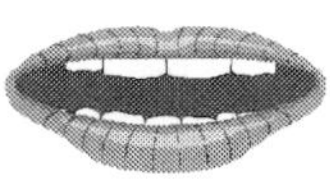

Solution:

29. knitting

puzzle

The written list was:

Cast-off, clustering, Fair-Isle, loops, pattern, ribbing, smocking, twist, welting, yarn.

The words can be matched to their respective initial lip-shapes in the following order.

1.
Fair-Isle,

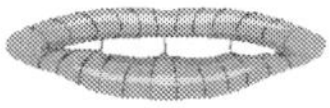

2.
loops,

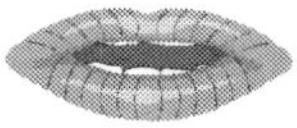

3.
twist,

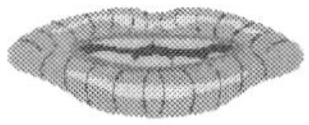

4.
smocking,

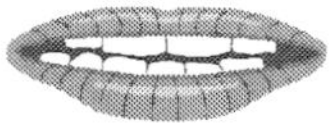

5.
pattern,

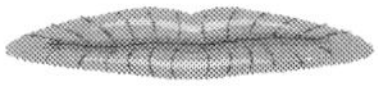

6.
welting,

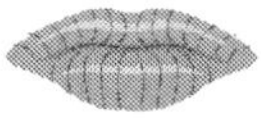

7.
clustering,

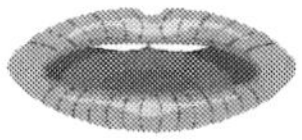

8.
ribbing,

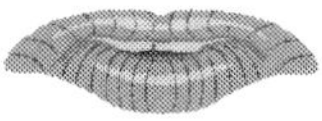

9.
yarn

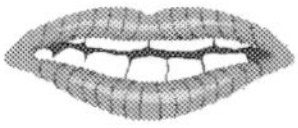

10.
Cast-off,

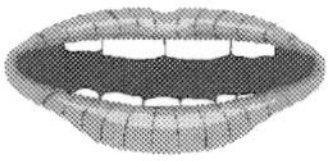

Lip-reading puzzle:

30. numbers

The pictures below represent **numbers** as a spoken list. The lip shape shown for each word is the first lip shape that would be seen by a lip-reader as the word is spoken.

Here are the words as a written list:
Quarter, half, one, two, four, six, eight, thirteen, hundred, million

Can you match the words on the list to the correct lip-shapes?

1.__________ 2.__________ 3.__________ 4.__________

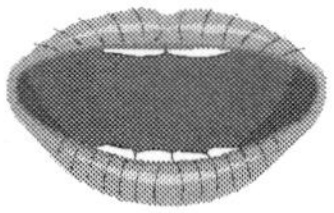
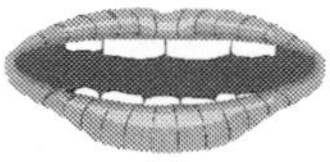
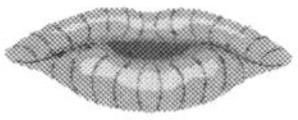
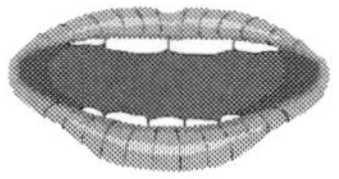

5.__________ 6.__________ 7.__________ 8.__________

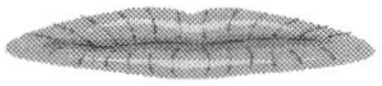
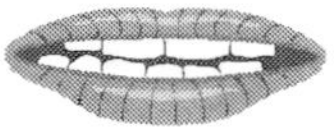
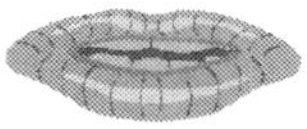
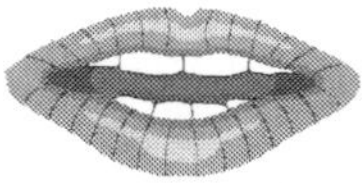

9.__________ 10.__________

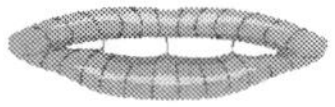
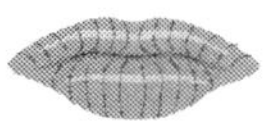

Solution:

30. numbers

puzzle

The written list was:

Quarter, half, one, two, four, six, eight, thirteen, hundred, million

The words can be matched to their respective initial lip-shapes in the following order.

1.
eight

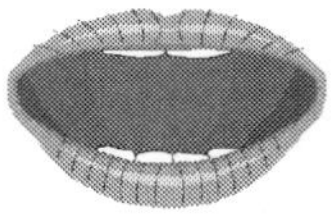

2.
half

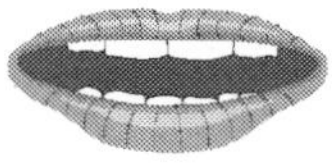

3.
quarter

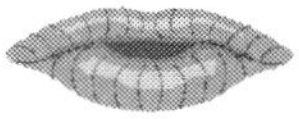

4.
hundred

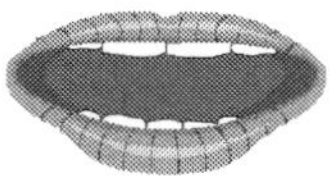

5.
million

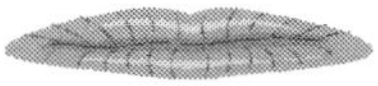

6.
six

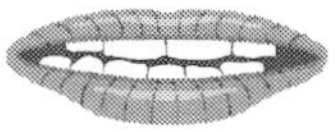

7.
two

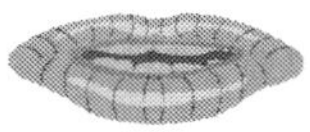

8.
thirteen

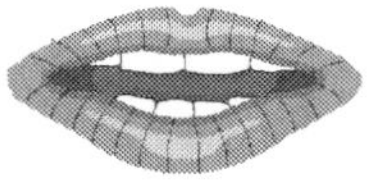

9.
four

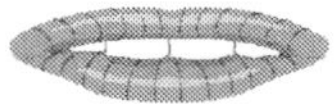

10.
one

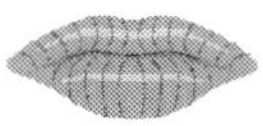

Lip-reading puzzle:

31. on the floor

words

The pictures below represent words about **flooring** as a spoken list. The lip shape shown for each is the first a lip-reader would see.

Here are the words as a written list:
Carpet, cleaning, gripper rods, length, mat, rug, stains, underlay, width, fitting.

Can you match the words on the list to the correct lip-shapes?

1.__________ 2.__________ 3.__________ 4.__________

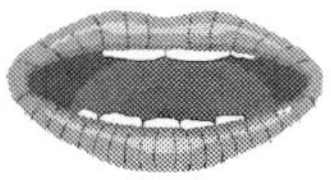
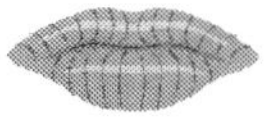
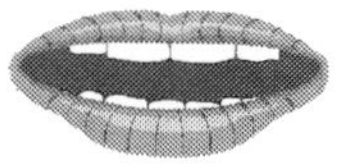
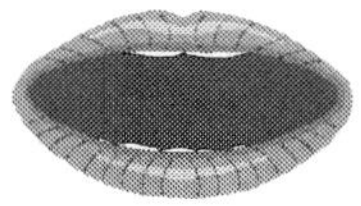

5.__________ 6.__________ 7.__________ 8.__________

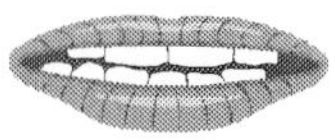
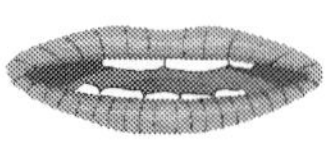
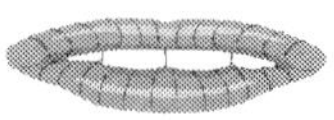
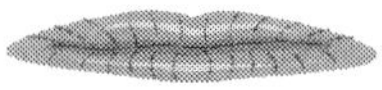

9.__________ 10.__________

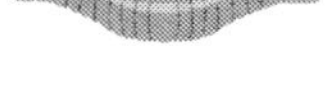
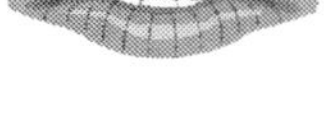

Solution:

31. on the floor

puzzle

The written list was:

Carpet, cleaning, gripper rods, length, mat, rug, stains, underlay, width, fitting.

The words can be matched to their respective initial lip-shapes in the following order.

1.
length

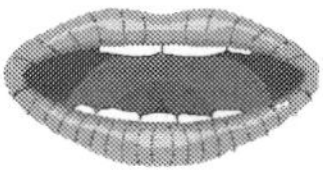

2.
width

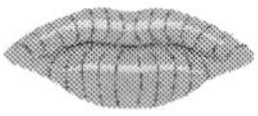

3.
carpet

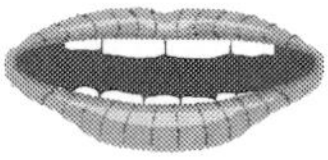

4.
underlay

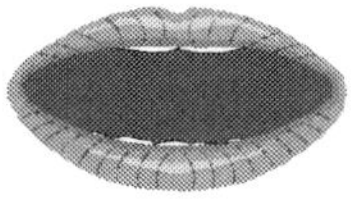

5.
stains

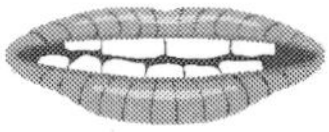

6.
cleaning

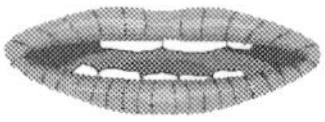

7.
fitting

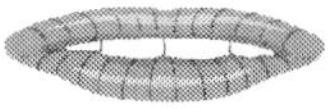

8.
mat

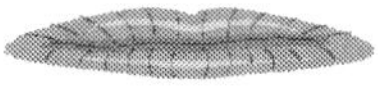

9.
rug

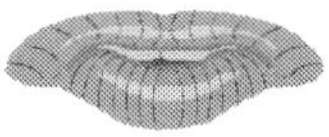

10.
gripper rods

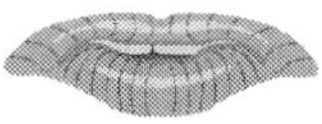

Lip-reading puzzle:

32. orienteering

The pictures below represent words to do with **orienteering** as a spoken list. The lip shape shown for each is the first lip shape a lip-reader would see.

Here are the words as a written list:
Clue sheet, compass, control point, map, navigation, orientation, route, short-cut, terrain, undergrowth, waypoint.

Can you match the words on the list to the correct lip-shapes?

1.__________ 2.__________ 3.__________ 4.__________

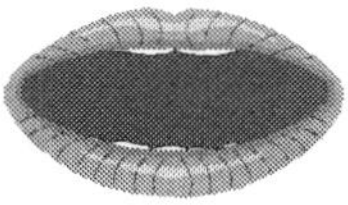
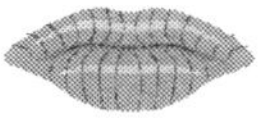
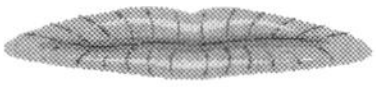
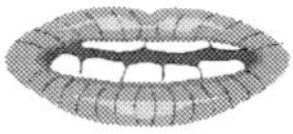

5.__________ 6.__________ 7.__________ 8.__________

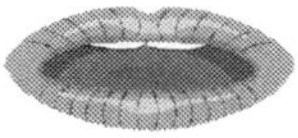
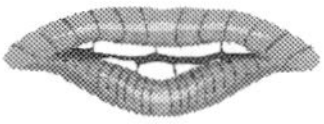
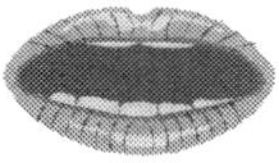
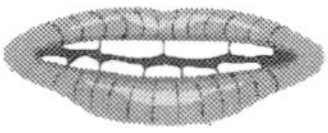

9.__________ 10.__________ 11.__________

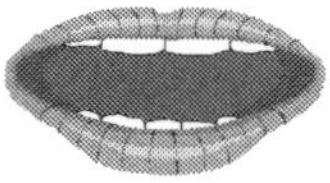
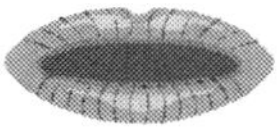
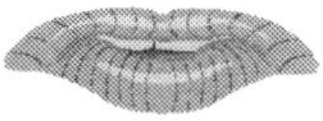

Solution:

32. orienteering

puzzle

The written list was:

Clue sheet, compass, control point, map, navigation, orientation, route, short-cut, terrain, undergrowth, waypoint.

The words can be matched to their respective initial lip-shapes in the following order.

1. undergrowth

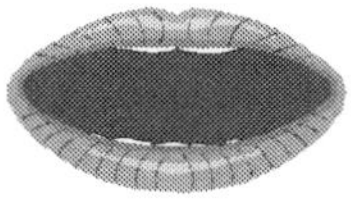

2. waypoint

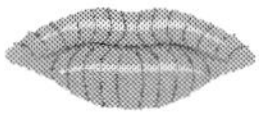

3. map

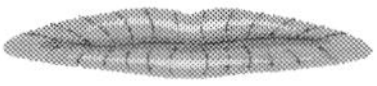

4. terrain

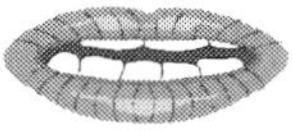

5. clue sheet

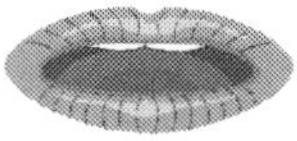

6. short-cut

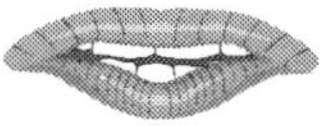

7. control point

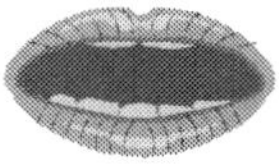

8. navigation

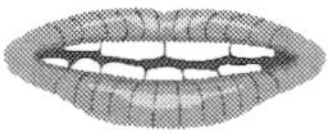

9. compass

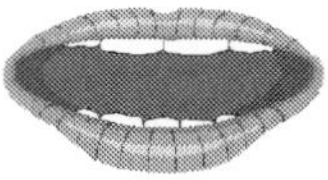

10. orientation

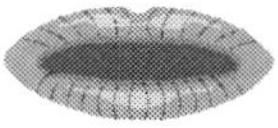

11. route

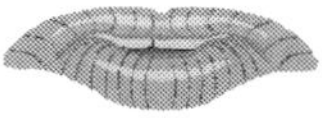

Lip-reading puzzle:

33. pathways

The pictures below represent words describing **pathways** as a spoken list. The lip shape shown for each word is the first lip shape that would be seen by a lip-reader as the word is spoken.

Here are the words as a written list:
Alley, course, esplanade, footpath, pavement, route, thoroughfare, tow-path, track, way.

Can you match the words on the list to the correct lip-shapes?

1.__________ 2.__________ 3.__________ 4.__________

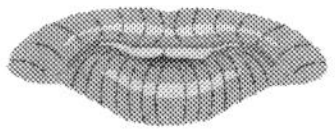
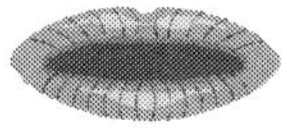
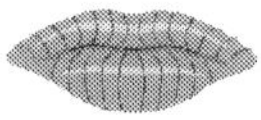
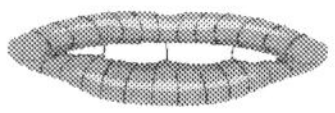

5.__________ 6.__________ 7.__________ 8.__________

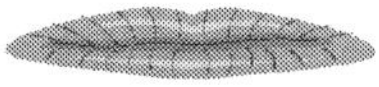
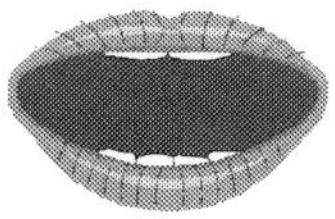
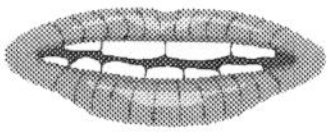
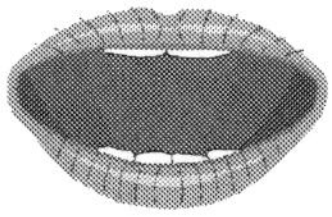

9.__________ 10.__________

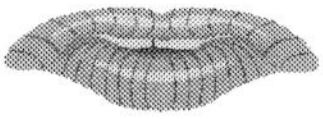
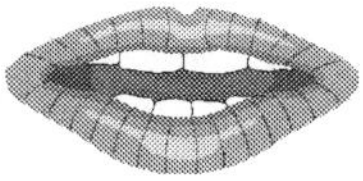

Solution:

33. pathways

puzzle

The written list was:
Alley, course, esplanade, footpath, pavement, route, thoroughfare, tow-path, track, way.

The words can be matched to their respective initial lip-shapes in the following order.

1.
track
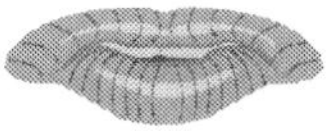

2.
course
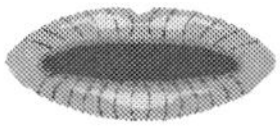

3.
way
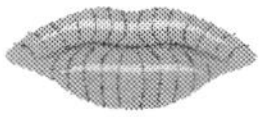

4.
footpath
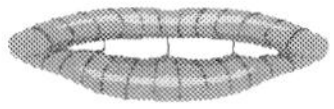

5.
pavement
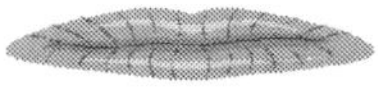

6.
alley
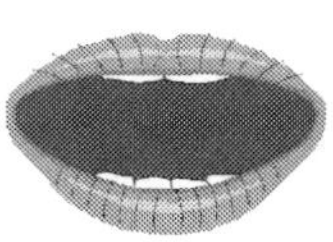

7.
tow-path
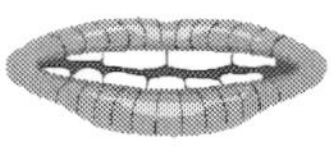

8.
esplanade
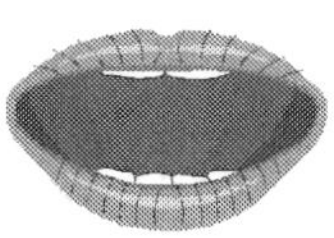

9.
route
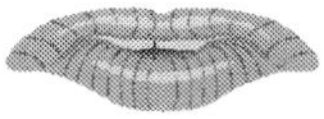

10.
thoroughfare
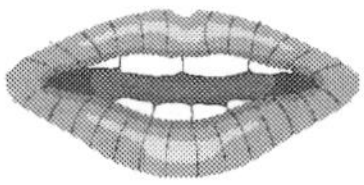

Lip-reading puzzle:

34. astronomy

The pictures below represent names of **planets and moons** as a spoken list. The lip shape shown for each name is the first seen by a lip-reader as the word is spoken.

Here are the names as a written list:
Io, Enceladus, Earth, Jupiter, Ganymede, Mercury, Neptune, Venus, Uranus.

Can you match the words on the list to the correct lip-shapes?

1.__________

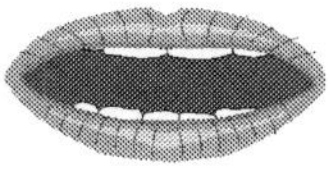

2.__________

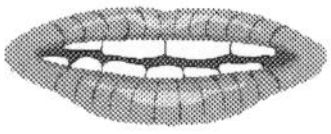

3.__________

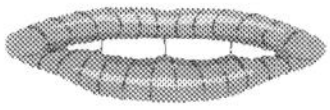

4.__________

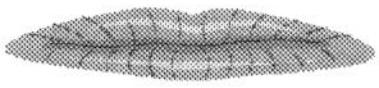

5.__________

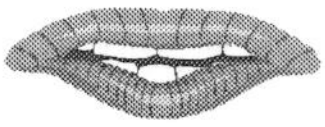

6.__________

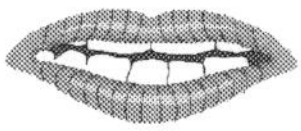

7.__________

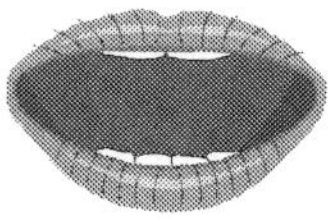

8.__________

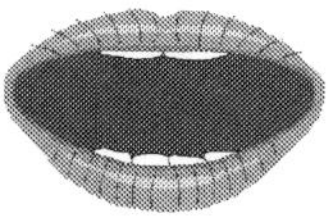

9.__________

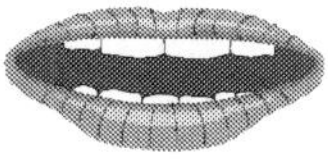

Solution:

34. astronomy

puzzle

The written list was:

Io, Enceladus, Earth, Jupiter, Ganymede, Mercury, Neptune, Venus, Uranus.

The words can be matched to their respective initial lip-shapes in the following order.

1. Earth

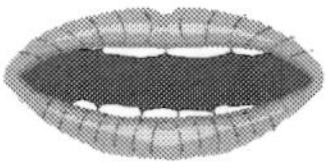

2. Neptune

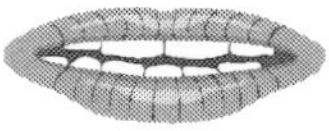

3. Venus

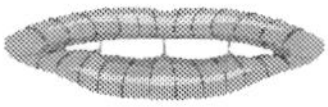

4. Mercury

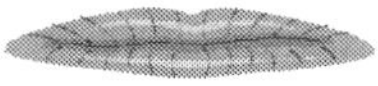

5. Jupiter

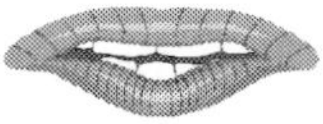

6. Uranus

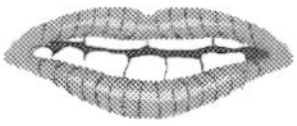

7. Enceladus

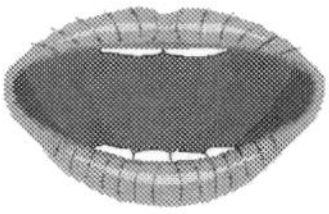

8. Io

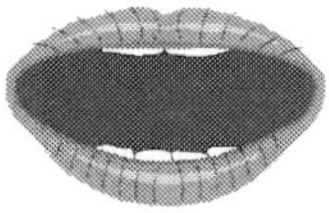

9. Ganymede

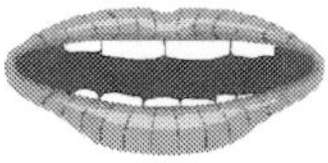

10.

11.

Lip-reading puzzle:

35. rail travel

The pictures below represent words associated with **rail travel** as a spoken list. The lip shape shown for each word is the first seen by a lip-reader.

Here are the words as a written list:
Electric train, junction, guard van, locomotive, monorail, off-peak fares, return ticket, dining car, freight train, one-way ticket.

Can you match the words on the list to the correct lip-shapes?

1.__________ 2.__________ 3.__________ 4.__________

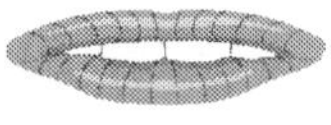
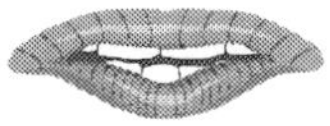
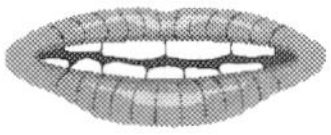
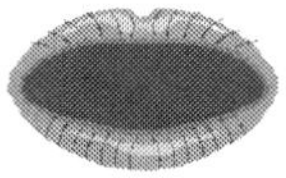

5.__________ 6.__________ 7.__________ 8.__________

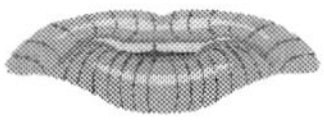
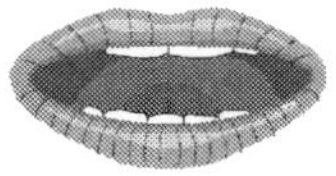
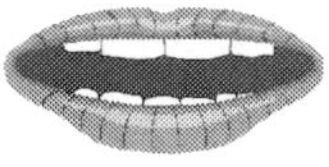
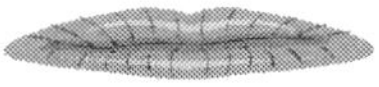

9.__________ 10.__________

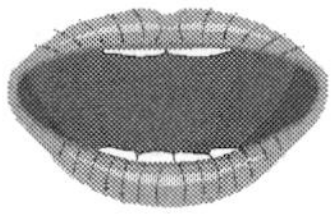
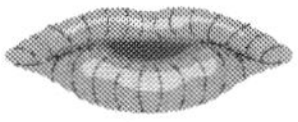

Solution:

35. rail travel

puzzle

The written list was:

Electric train, junction, guard van, locomotive, monorail, off-peak fares, return ticket, dining car, freight train, one-way ticket.

The words can be matched to their respective initial lip-shapes in the following order.

1.
freight train

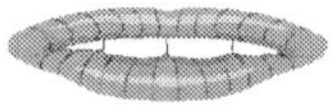

2.
junction

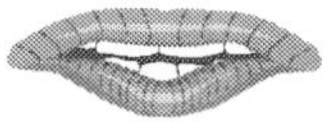

3.
dining car

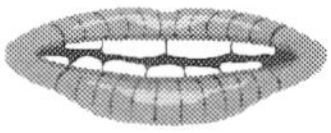

4.
off-peak fares

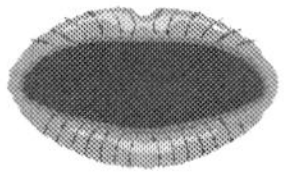

5.
return ticket

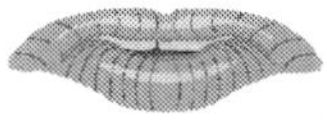

6.
locomotive

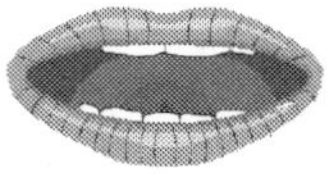

7.
Guard van

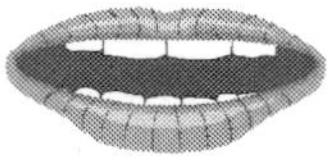

8.
monorail

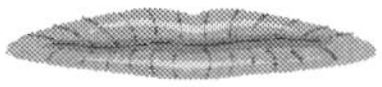

9.
electric train

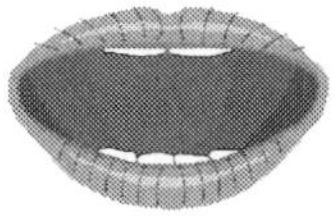

10.
one-way ticket

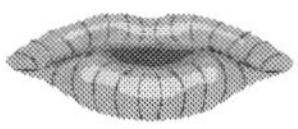

Lip-reading puzzle:

36. roads

The pictures below represent words to do with **road conditions** as a spoken list. The lip shape shown for each word is the first seen by a lip-reader.

Here are the words as a written list:
Winding, pot-hole, congestion, traffic control, hard-shoulder, overtaking, visibility, dazzle, lighting, junction, zone.

Can you match the words on the list to the correct lip-shapes?

1.__________ 2.__________ 3.__________ 4.__________

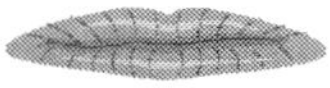
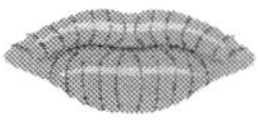
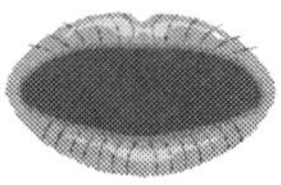
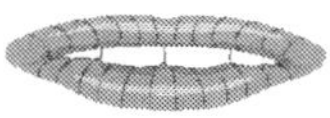

5.__________ 6.__________ 7.__________ 8.__________

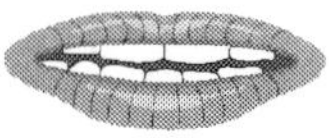
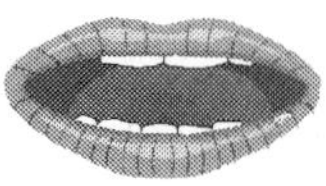
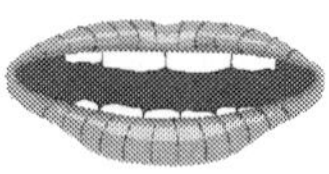
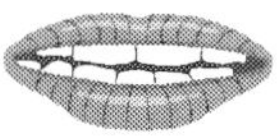

9.__________ 10.__________ 11.__________

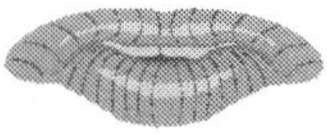
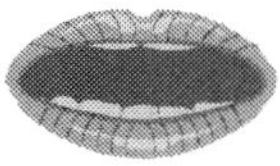
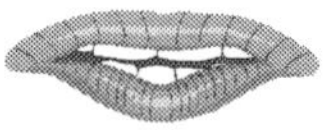

Solution:

36. roads

puzzle

The written list was:

Winding, pot-hole, congestion, traffic control, hard-shoulder, overtaking, visibility, dazzle, lighting, junction, zone.

The words can be matched to their respective initial lip-shapes in the following order.

1. pot-hole

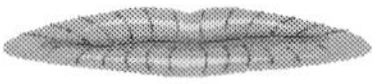

2. winding

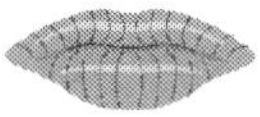

3. overtaking

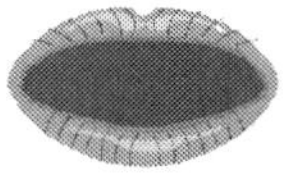

4. visibility

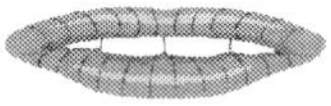

5. dazzle

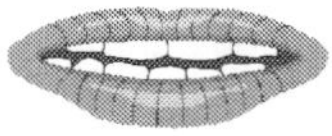

6. lighting

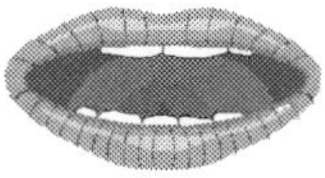

7. hard-shoulder

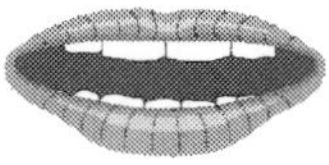

8. zone

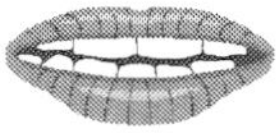

9. traffic control

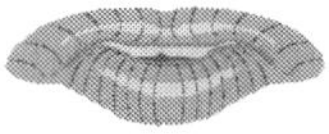

10. congestion

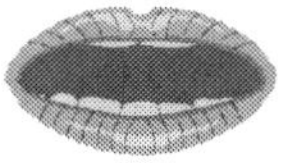

11. junction

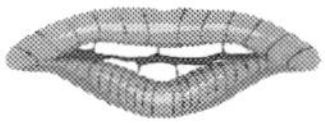

Lip-reading puzzle:

37. lessons

The pictures below represent names of **school subjects** as a spoken list. The lip shape shown for each is the first a lip-reader would see.

Here are the words as a written list:
Engineering, geography, chemistry, history, crafts, cookery, library studies, biology, rural science, science, physics, woodwork.

Can you match the words on the list to the correct lip-shapes?

1.__________ 2.__________ 3.__________ 4.__________

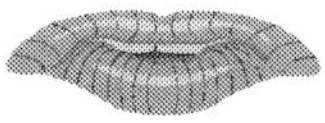
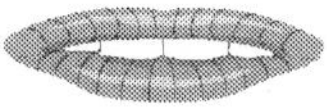
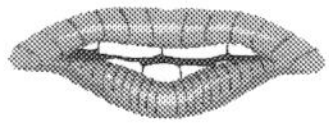
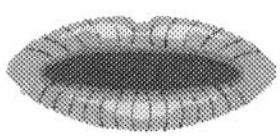

5.__________ 6.__________ 7.__________ 8.__________

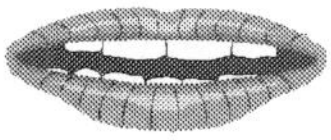
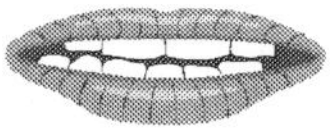
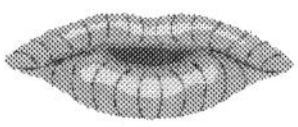
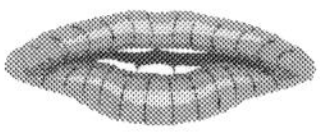

9.__________ 10.__________ 11.__________ 12.__________

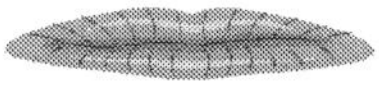
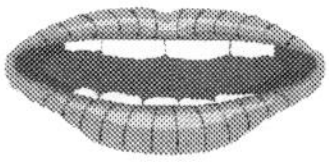
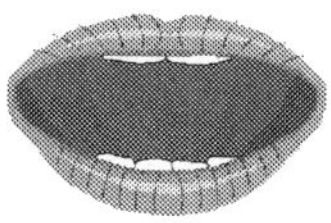
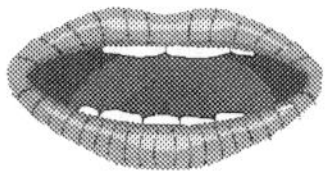

Solution:

37. lessons

puzzle

The written list was:

Engineering, geography, chemistry, history, crafts, cookery, library studies, biology, rural science, science, physics, woodwork.

The words can be matched to their respective initial lip-shapes in the following order.

1. rural science

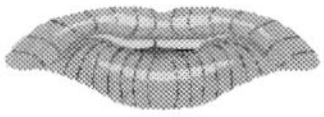

2. physics

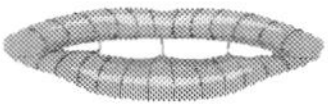

3. geography

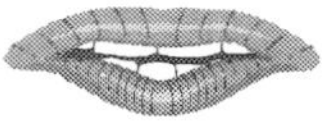

4. cookery

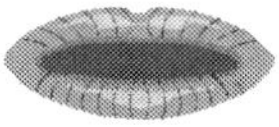

5. history

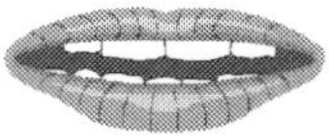

6. science

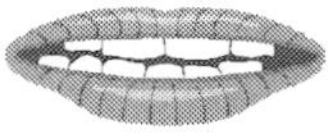

7. woodwork

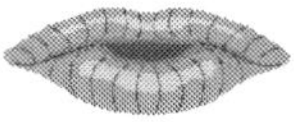

8. crafts

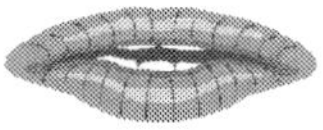

9. biology

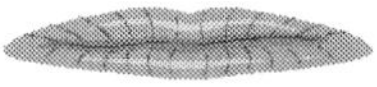

10. chemistry

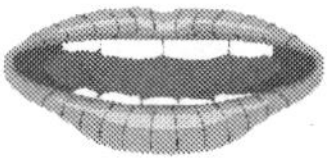

11. engineering

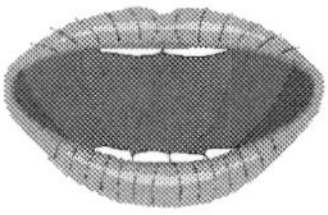

12. library studies

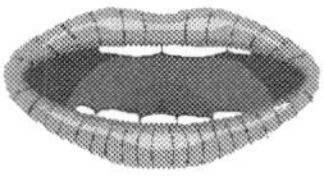

Lip-reading puzzle:

38. school

The pictures below represent words to do with **school** as a spoken list. The lip shape shown for each word is the first a lip reader would see.

Here are the words as a written list:
Exercise book, fire practice, games, goal post, gymnasium, lesson, playground, ruler, teacher, white board.

Can you match the words on the list to the correct lip-shapes?

1.__________

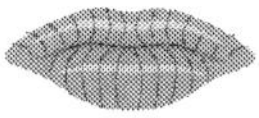

2.__________

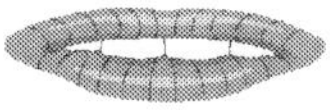

3.__________

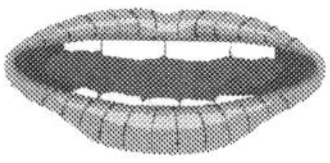

4.__________

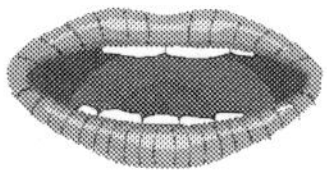

5.__________

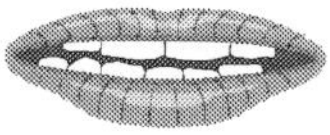

6.__________

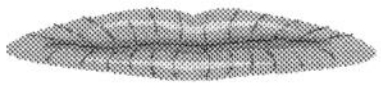

7.__________

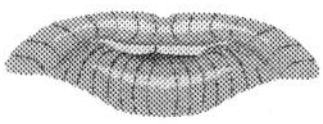

8.__________

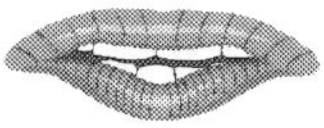

9.__________

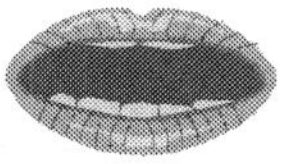

10.__________

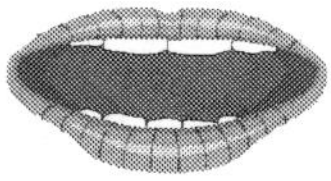

Solution:

38. school

puzzle

The written list was:

Exercise book, fire practice, games, goal post, gymnasium, lesson, playground, ruler, teacher, white board.

The words can be matched to their respective initial lip-shapes in the following order.

1. white board

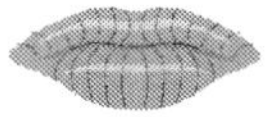

2. fire practice

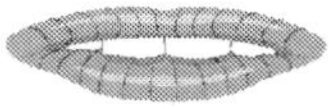

3. games

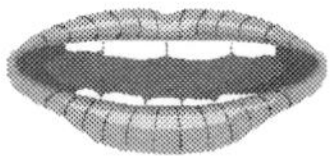

4. lesson

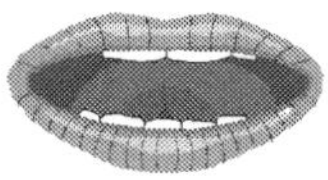

5. teacher

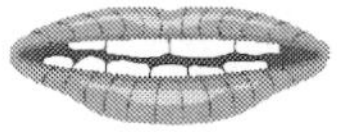

6. playground

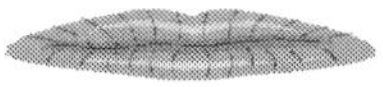

7. ruler

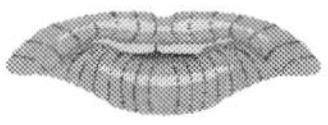

8. gymnasium

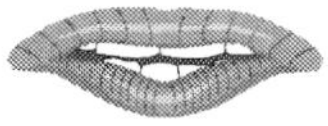

9. goal post

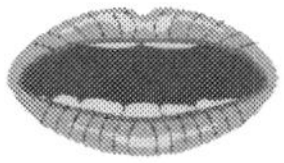

10. exercise book

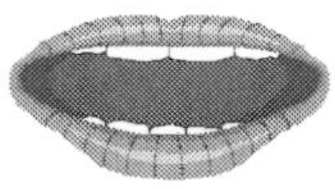

11.

12.

Lip-reading puzzle:

39. sea fish

The pictures below represent names of **sea fish** as a spoken list. The lip shape shown for each word is the first lip shape that would be seen by a lip-reader as the word is spoken.

Here are the words as a written list:
Halibut, Hake, Cod, Lemon sole, Mackerel, Turbot, Tiddler, Tuna, Flounder, Whiting.
Can you match the words on the list to the correct lip-shapes?

1.__________

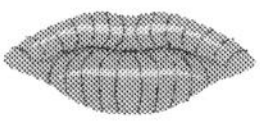

2.__________

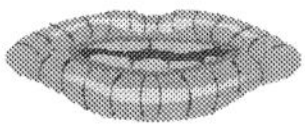

3.__________

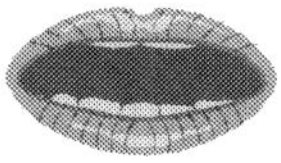

4.__________

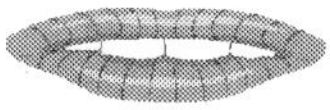

5.__________

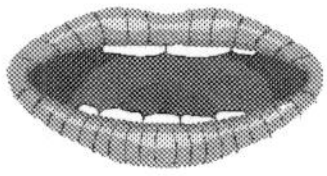

6.__________

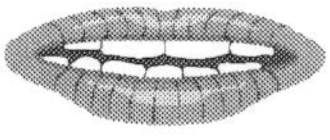

7.__________

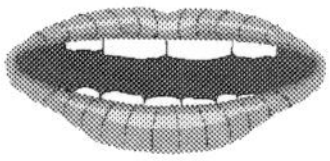

8.__________

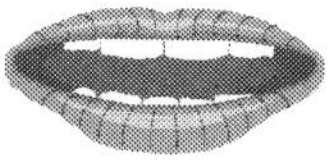

9.__________

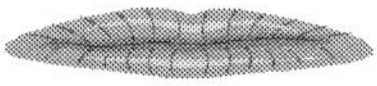

10.__________

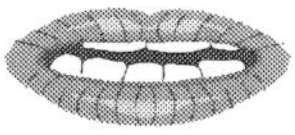

Solution:

39. sea fish

puzzle

The written list was:
Halibut, Hake, Cod, Lemon sole, Mackerel, Turbot, Tiddler, Tuna, Flounder, Whiting.

The words can be matched to their respective initial lip-shapes in the following order.

1.
Whiting

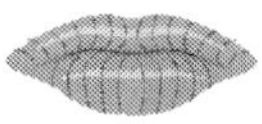

2.
Tuna

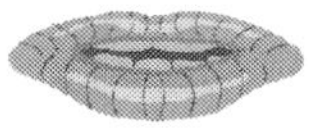

3.
Cod

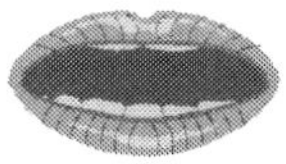

4.
Flounder

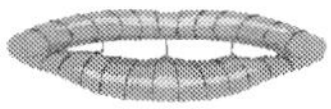

5.
Lemon sole

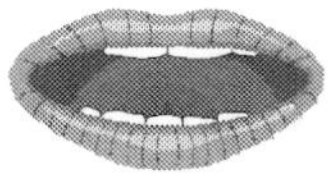

6.
Tiddler

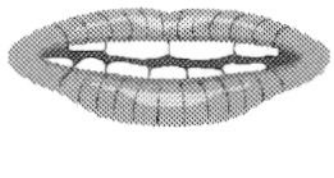

7.
Halibut

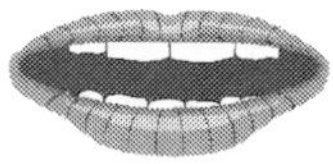

8.
Hake

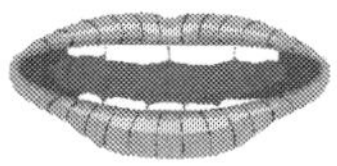

9.
Mackerel

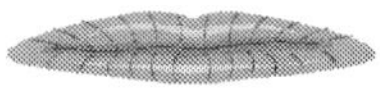

10.
Turbot

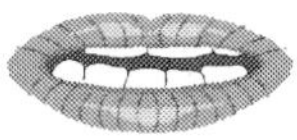

Lip-reading puzzle:

40. sea shore

The pictures below represent things to be seen on the **sea shore** as a spoken list. The lip shape shown for each word is the first lip shape that would be seen by a lip-reader as the word is spoken.

Here are the words as a written list:
Shells, hermit crab, horizon, gravel, lifebuoy, breakers, rocks, seaweed, dune, flotsam, waves

Can you match the words on the list to the correct lip-shapes?

1.__________ 2.__________ 3.__________ 4.__________

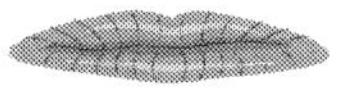
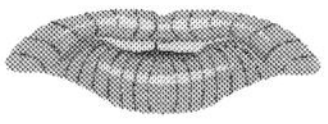
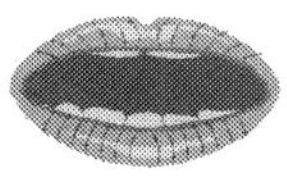
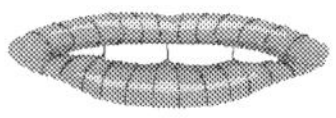

5.__________ 6.__________ 7.__________ 8.__________

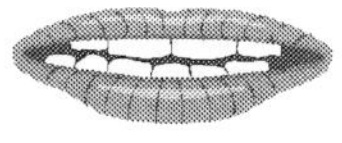
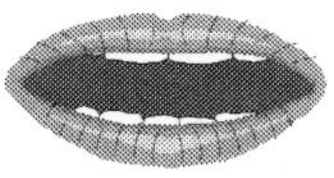
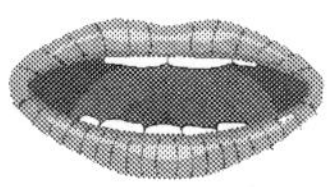
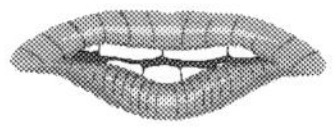

9.__________ 10.__________ 11.__________

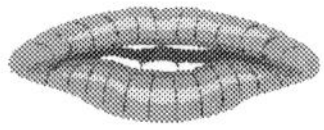
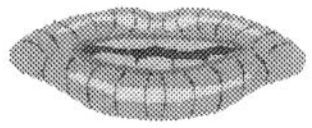
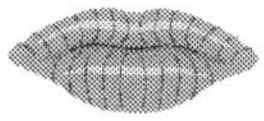

Solution:

40. sea shore

puzzle

The written list was:

Shells, hermit crab, horizon, gravel, lifebuoy, breakers, rocks, seaweed, dune, flotsam, waves

The words can be matched to their respective initial lip-shapes in the following order.

1.
breakers

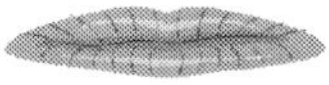

2.
rocks

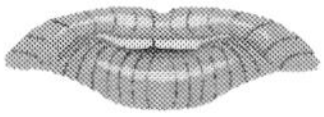

3.
horizon

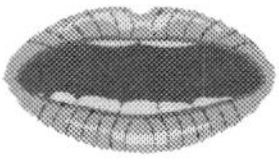

4.
flotsam

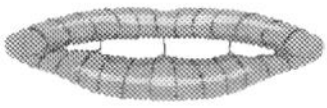

5.
seaweed

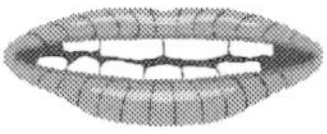

6.
hermit crab

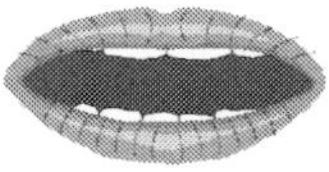

7.
lifebuoy

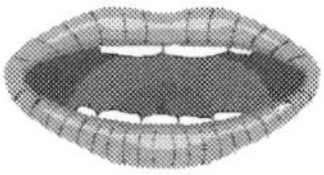

8.
shells

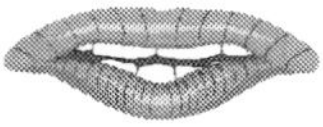

9.
gravel

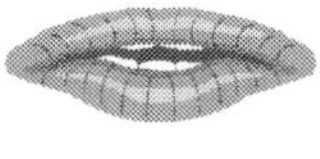

10.
dune

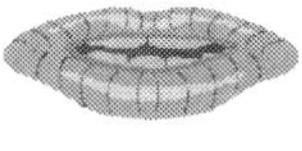

11.
waves

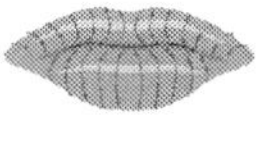

Lip-reading puzzle:

41. seating

The pictures below represent words to do with **seating** as a spoken list. The lip shape shown for each word is the first seen by a lip-reader.

Here are the words as a written list:
Armchair, chair, high chair, leather chair, bench, office chair, rocking chair, deckchair, wicker chair, throne.

Can you match the words on the list to the correct lip-shapes?

1.__________ 2.__________ 3.__________ 4.__________

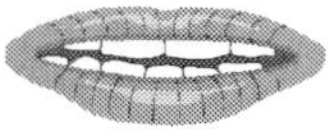
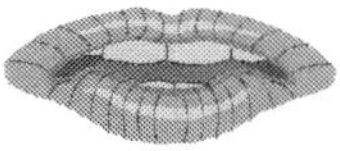
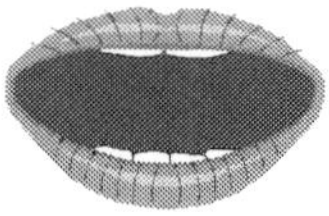
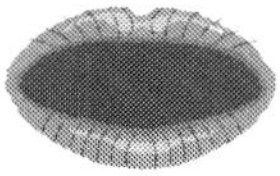

5.__________ 6.__________ 7.__________ 8.__________

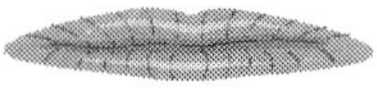
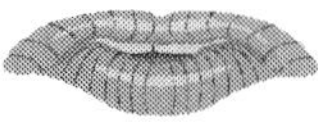
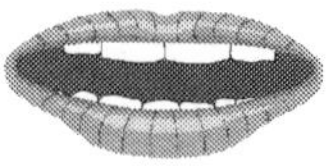
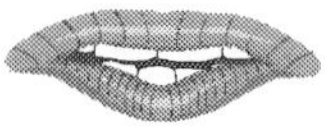

9.__________ 10.__________

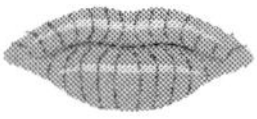
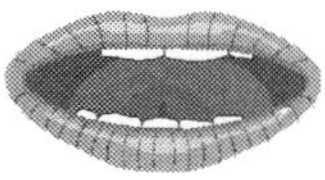

Solution:

41. seating

puzzle

The written list was:

Armchair, chair, high chair, leather chair, bench, office chair, rocking chair, deckchair, wicker chair, throne.

The words can be matched to their respective initial lip-shapes in the following order.

1. deckchair

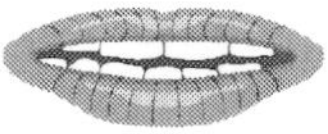

2. throne

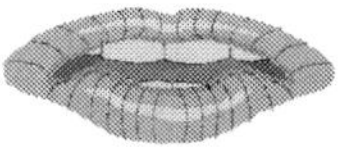

3. armchair

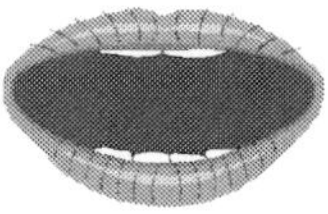

4. office chair

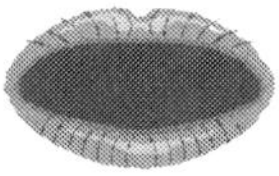

5. bench

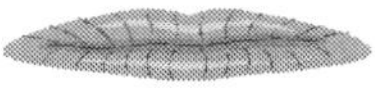

6. rocking chair

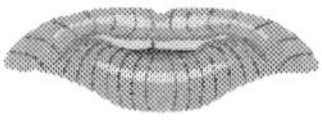

7. high chair

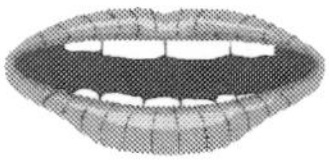

8. chair

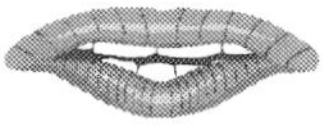

9. wicker chair

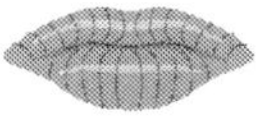

10. leather chair

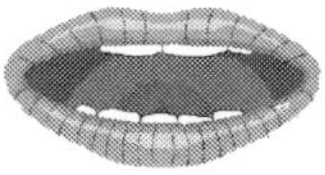

11.

12.

Lip-reading puzzle:

42. shopping list

The pictures below represent items written on my **shopping list** as a spoken list. The lip shape shown for each item is the first lip shape that would be seen by a lip-reader as the word is spoken.

Here are the words as a written list:
Butter, custard, figs, jelly, lemons, radishes, thread, tea bags, washing powder.

Can you match the words on the list to the correct lip-shapes?

1.__________ 2.__________ 3.__________ 4.__________

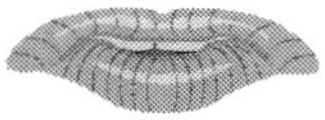 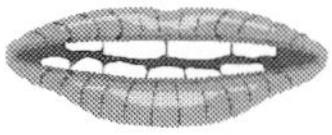 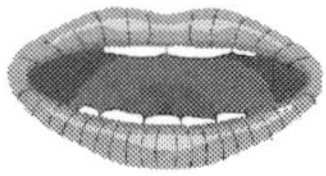 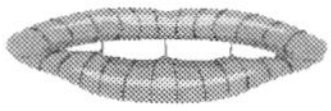

5.__________ 6.__________ 7.__________ 8.__________

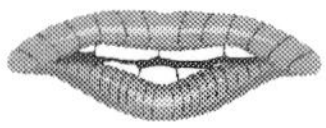 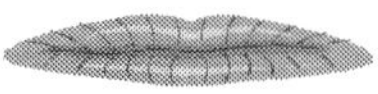 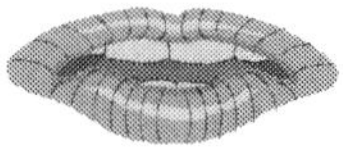 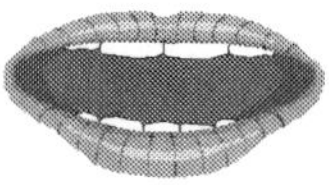

9.__________

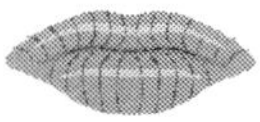

Solution:

42. shopping list

puzzle

The written list was:

Butter, custard, figs, jelly, lemons, radishes, thread, tea bags, washing powder.

The words can be matched to their respective initial lip-shapes in the following order.

1. radishes

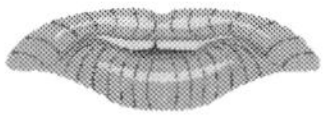

2. tea bags

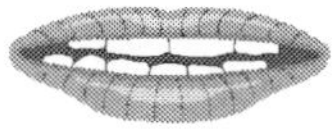

3. lemons

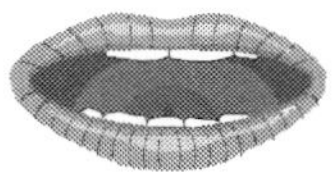

4. figs

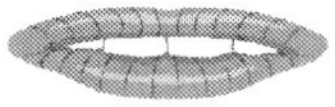

5. jelly

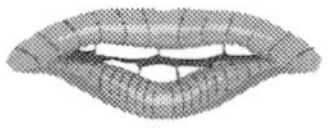

6. butter

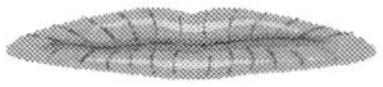

7. thread

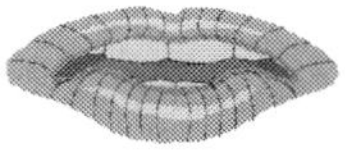

8. custard

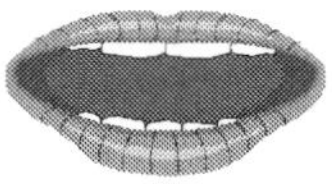

9. washing powder

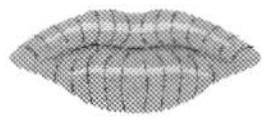

Lip-reading puzzle:

43. skiing

The pictures below represent words to do with **skiing** as a spoken list. The lip shape shown for each word is the first lip shape that would be seen by a lip-reader as the word is spoken.

Here are the words as a written list:
Alpine, chair-lift, helmet, gloves, cross-country, goggles, boots, snowboard, Nordic, free-style.
Can you match the words on the list to the correct lip-shapes?

1.__________ 2.__________ 3.__________ 4.__________

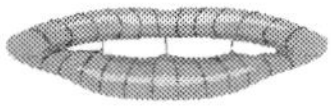
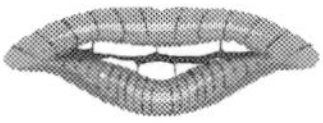
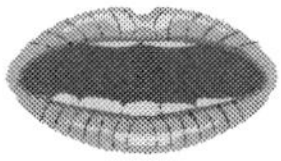
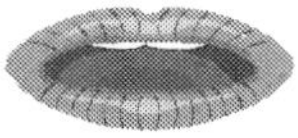

5.__________ 6.__________ 7.__________ 8.__________

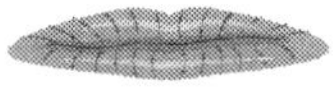
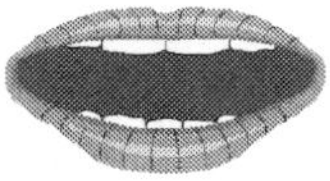
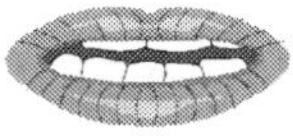
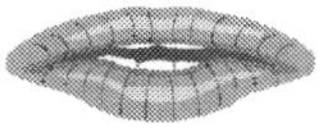

9.__________ 10.__________

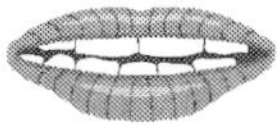
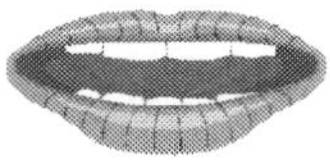

Solution:

43. skiing

puzzle

The written list was:

Alpine, chair-lift, helmet, gloves, cross-country, goggles, boots, snowboard, Nordic, free-style.

The words can be matched to their respective initial lip-shapes in the following order.

1. free-style

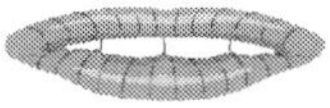

2. chair-lift

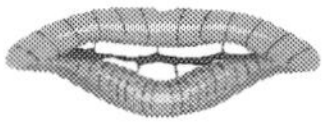

3. goggles

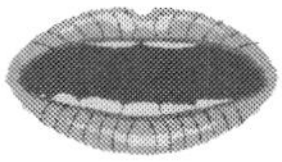

4. gloves

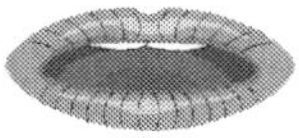

5. boots

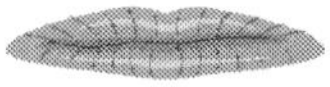

6. alpine

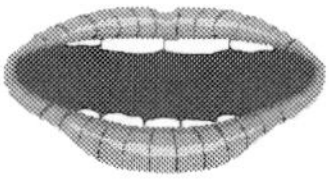

7. Nordic

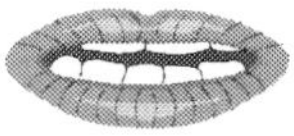

8. cross-country

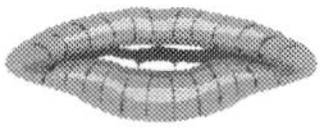

9. snowboard

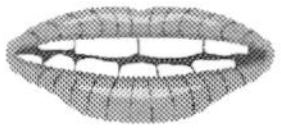

10. helmet

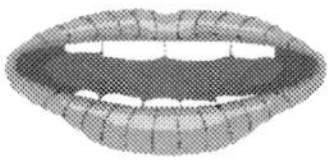

Lip-reading puzzle:

44. stationery

The pictures below represent words to do with **stationery** as a spoken list. The lip shape shown for each word is the first lip shape that would be seen by a lip-reader as the word is spoken.

Here are the words as a written list:
Eraser, pencil, highlighter, clips, stapler, shredder, folder, ring binder, loose leaf, wallet, crayons.

Can you match the words on the list to the correct lip-shapes?

1.__________

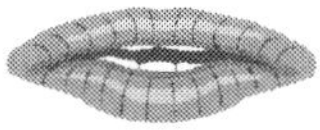

2.__________

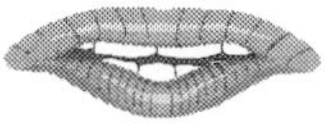

3.__________

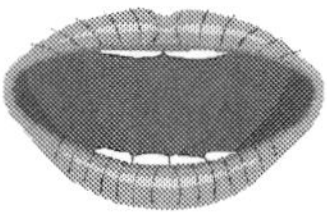

4.__________

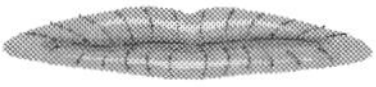

5.__________

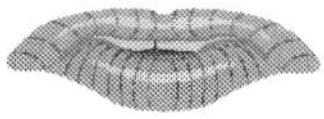

6.__________

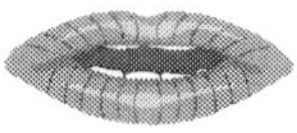

7.__________

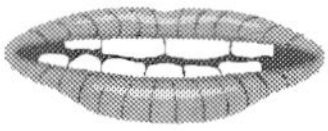

8.__________

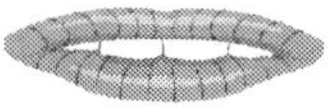

9.__________

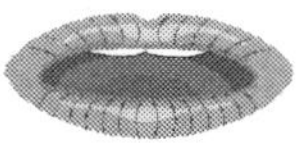

10.__________

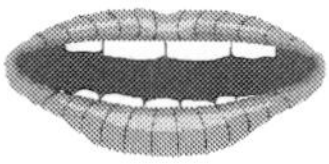

11.__________

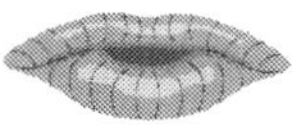

Solution:

44. stationery

puzzle

The written list was:

Eraser, pencil, highlighter, clips, stapler, shredder, folder, ring binder, loose leaf, wallet, crayons.

The words can be matched to their respective initial lip-shapes in the following order.

1.
crayons

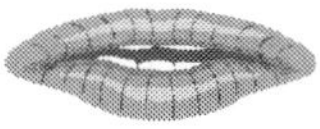

2.
shredder

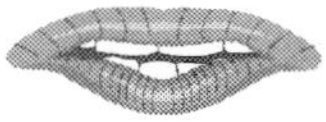

3.
eraser

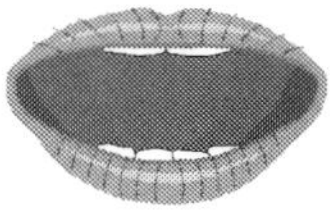

4.
pencil

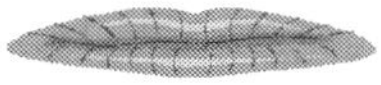

5.
ring binder

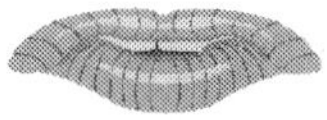

6.
loose leaf

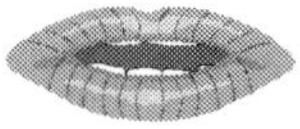

7.
stapler

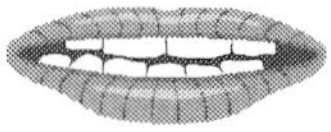

8.
folder

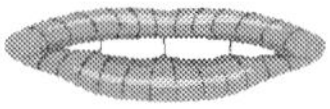

9.
clips

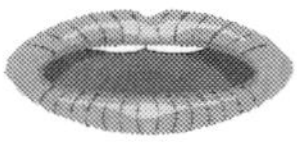

10.
highlighter

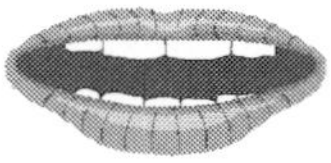

11.
wallet

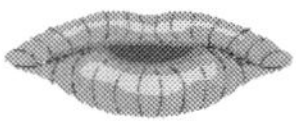

Lip reading puzzle:

45. TV quizzes

The pictures below represent words to do with **TV quizzes** as a spoken list. The lip shape shown for each word is the first lip shape that would be seen by a lip-reader as the word is spoken.

Here are the words as a written list:
Questions, answers, easy, choices, higher, lower, looser, prizes, score, winner.

Can you match the words on the list to the correct lip-shapes?

1.__________ 2.__________ 3.__________ 4.__________

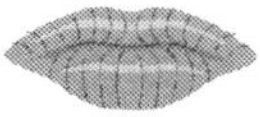
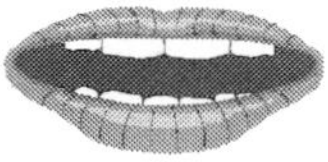
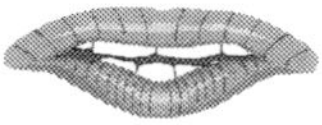
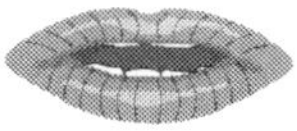

5.__________ 6.__________ 7.__________ 8.__________

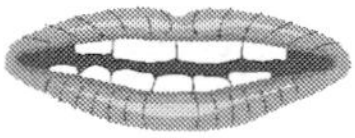
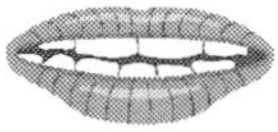
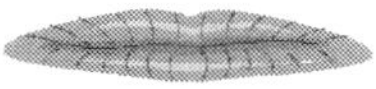
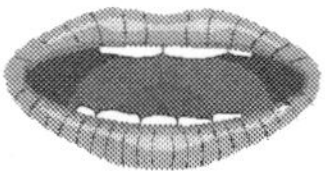

9.__________ 10.__________

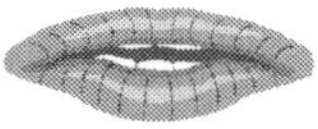
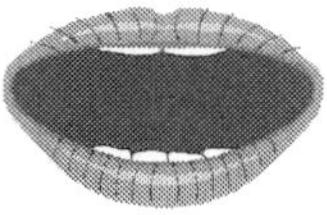

Solution:

45. TV quizzes

puzzle

The written list was:

Questions, answers, easy, choices, higher, lower, looser, prizes, score, winner.

The words can be matched to their respective initial lip-shapes in the following order.

1. winner

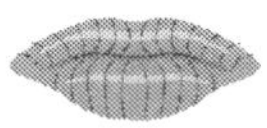

2. higher

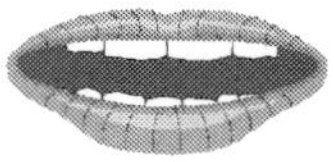

3. choices

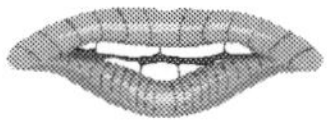

4. looser

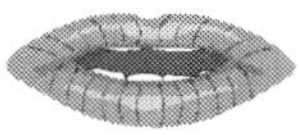

5. easy

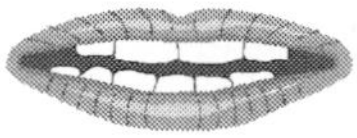

6. score

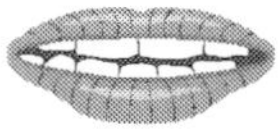

7. prizes

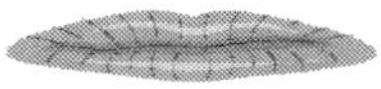

8. lower

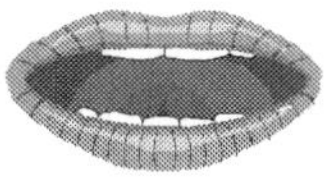

9. question

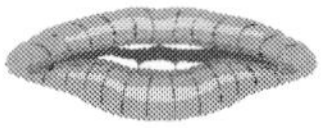

10. answers

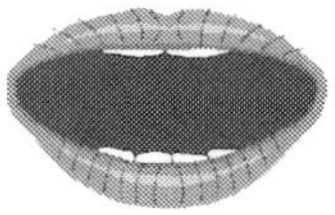

Lip-reading puzzle:

46. types of mill

The pictures below represent words describing **types of mill** as a spoken list. The lip shape shown is the first seen by a lip-reader as the word is spoken.

Here are the words as a written list:
Hammer mill, coffee mill, grinding mill, corn mill, paper mill, roller mill, sawmill, treadmill, windmill, vertical mill.
Can you match the words on the list to the correct lip-shapes?

1.__________ 2.__________ 3.__________ 4.__________

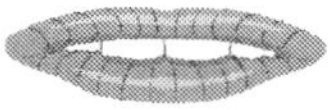 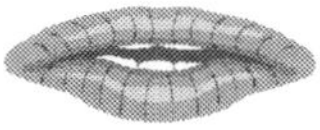 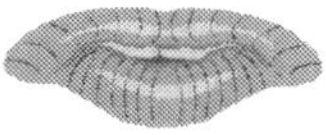 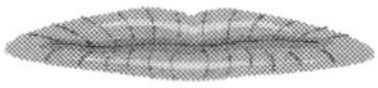

5.__________ 6.__________ 7.__________ 8.__________

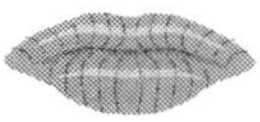 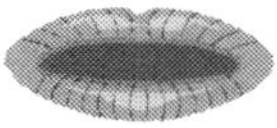 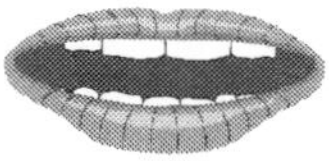 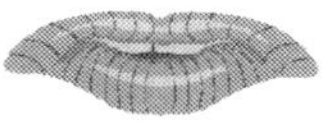

9.__________ 10.__________

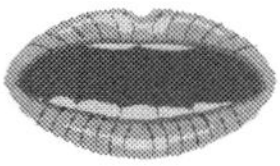 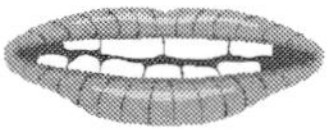

Solution:

46. types of mill

puzzle

The written list was:

Hammer mill, coffee mill, grinding mill, corn mill, paper mill, roller mill, sawmill, treadmill, windmill, vertical mill.

The words can be matched to their respective initial lip-shapes in the following order.

1. vertical mill

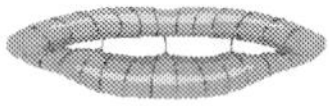

2. grinding mill

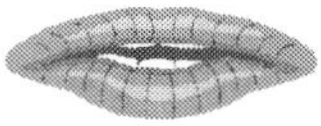

3. treadmill

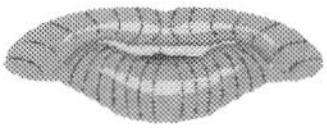

4. paper mill

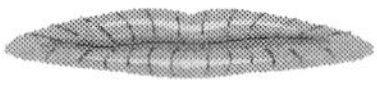

5. windmill

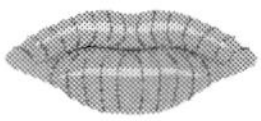

6. corn mill

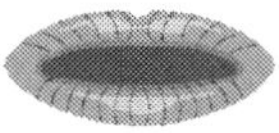

7. hammer mill

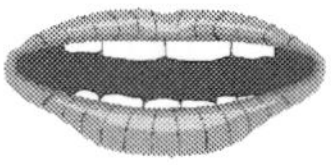

8. roller mill

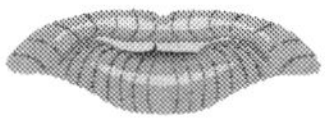

9. coffee mill

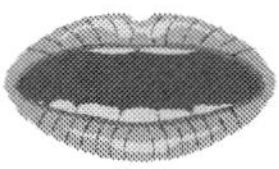

10. sawmill

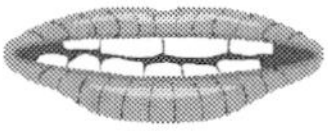

Lip-reading puzzle:

47. vineyards

The pictures below represent words to do with **vineyards** as a spoken list. The lip shape shown for each is the first seen by a lip-reader when the word is spoken.

Here are the words as a written list:
Vines, grapes, blossom, weeding, sunshine, ripening, labelling, corks, thinning, choosing.

Can you match the words on the list to the correct lip-shapes?

1.____________ 2.____________ 3.____________ 4.____________

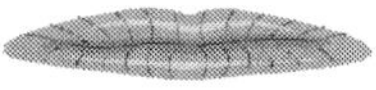
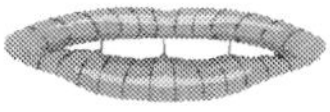
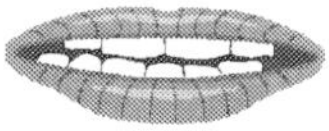
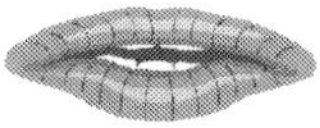

5.____________ 6.____________ 7.____________ 8.____________

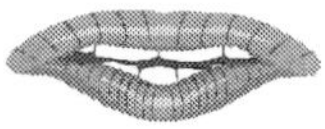
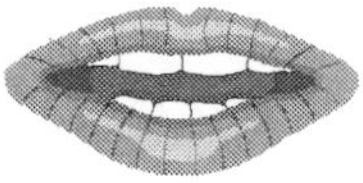
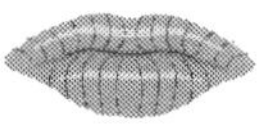
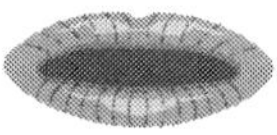

9.____________ 10.____________

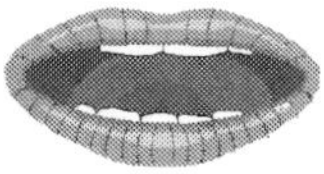
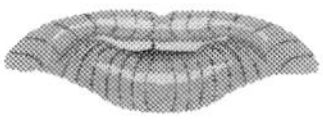

Solution:

47. vineyards

puzzle

The written list was:

Vines, grapes, blossom, weeding, sunshine, ripening, labelling, corks, thinning, choosing.

The words can be matched to their respective initial lip-shapes in the following order.

1.
blossom

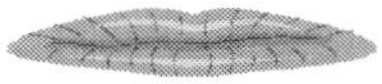

2.
vines

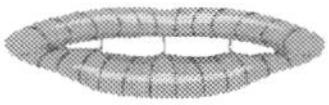

3.
sunshine

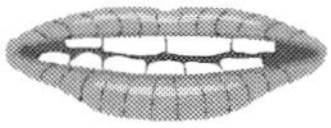

4.
grapes

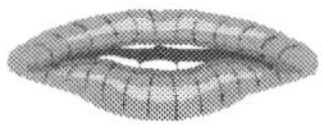

5.
choosing

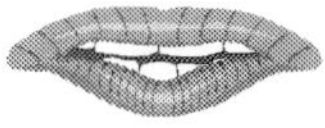

6.
thinning

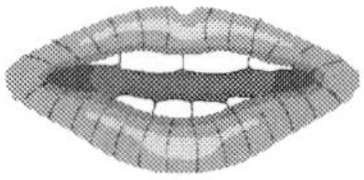

7.
weeding

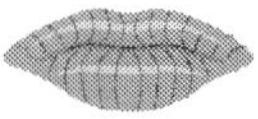

8.
corks

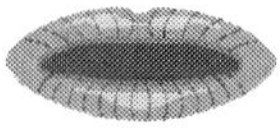

9.
labelling

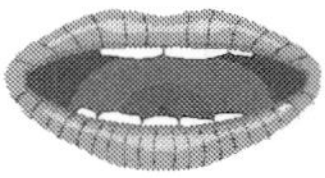

10.
ripening

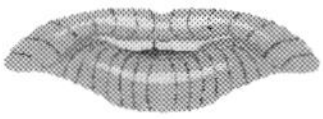

Lip-reading puzzle:

48. weather

The pictures below represent words describing features of **weather** as a spoken list. The lip shape shown for each word is the first lip shape that would be seen by a lip-reader as the word is spoken.

Here are the words as a written list:
Lightning, overcast, rain, sunshine, thunder, hail, ultra-violet, frost, wind, ice, clouds.

Can you match the words on the list to the correct lip-shapes?

1.__________

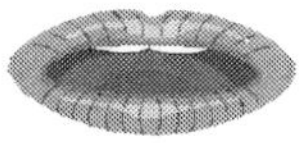

2.__________

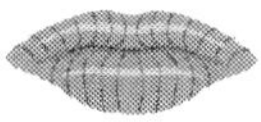

3.__________

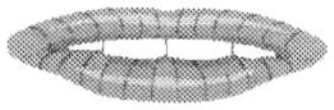

4.__________

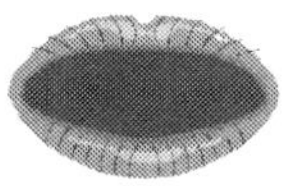

5.__________

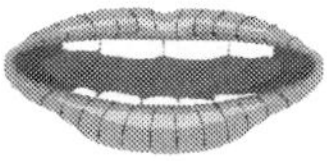

6.__________

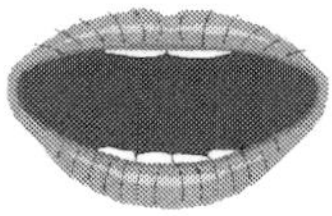

7.__________

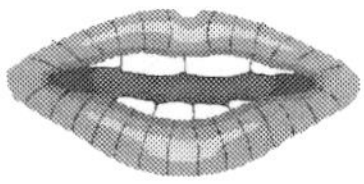

8.__________

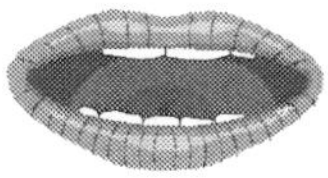

9.__________

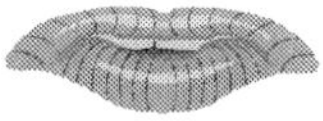

10.__________

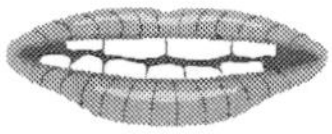

11.__________

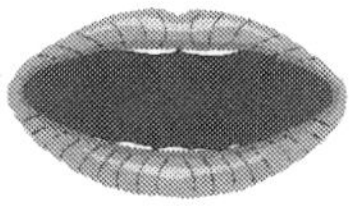

Solution:

48. weather

puzzle

The written list was:

Lightning, overcast, rain, sunshine, thunder, hail, ultra-violet, frost, wind, ice, clouds.

The words can be matched to their respective initial lip-shapes in the following order.

1\. clouds

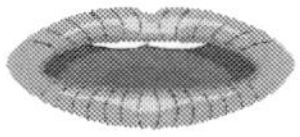

2\. wind

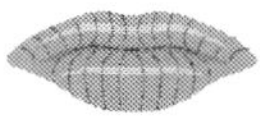

3\. frost

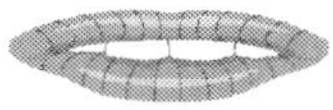

4\. overcast

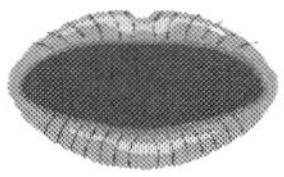

5\. hail

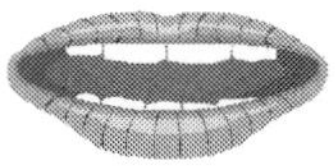

6\. ice

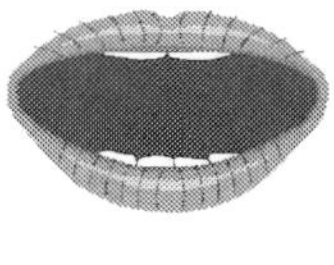

7\. thunder

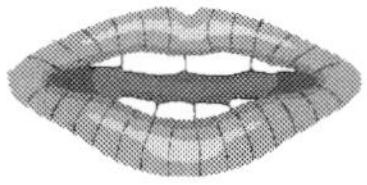

8\. lightning

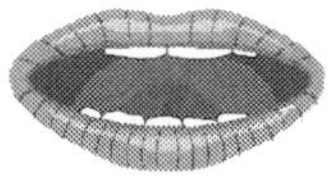

9\. rain

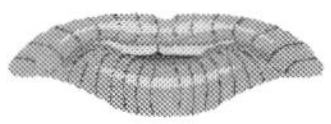

10\. sunshine

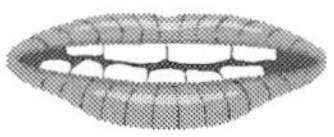

11\. ultra-violet

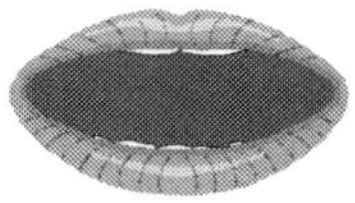

Lip-reading puzzle:

49. windows

The pictures below represent words describing **window types** as a spoken list. The lip shape shown for each word is the first lip shape that would be seen by a lip-reader as the word is spoken.

Here are the words as a written list:
Casement, hopper, cross, lantern, bay, skylight, transom, thermal, oriel, French.

Can you match the words on the list to the correct lip-shapes?

1.__________

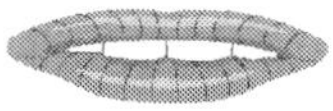

2.__________

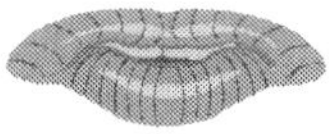

3.__________

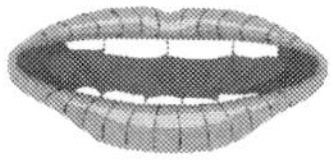

4.__________

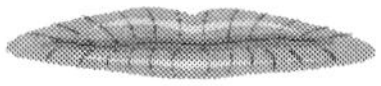

5.__________

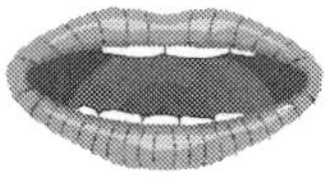

6.__________

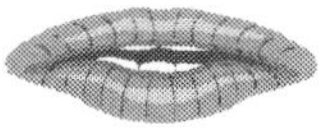

7.__________

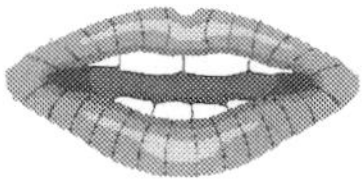

8.__________

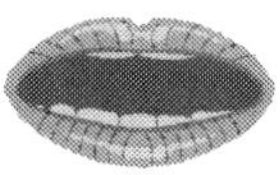

9.__________

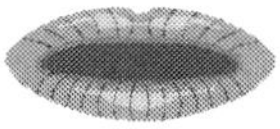

10.__________

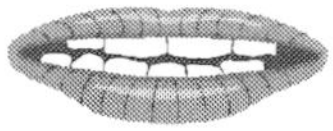

Solution:

49. windows

puzzle

The written list was:

Casement, hopper, cross, lantern, bay, skylight, transom, thermal, oriel, French.

The words can be matched to their respective initial lip-shapes in the following order.

1. French

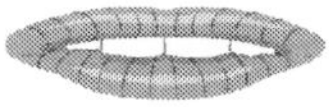

2. transom

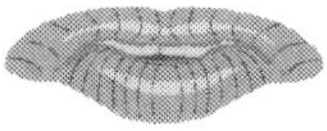

3. casement

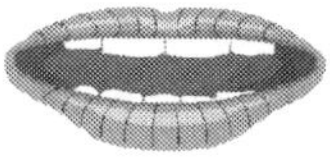

4. bay

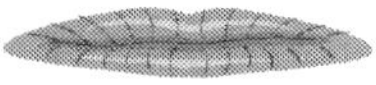

5. lantern

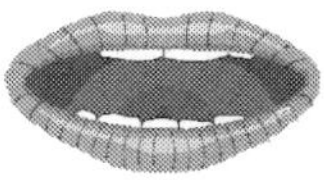

6. cross

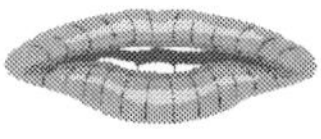

7. thermal

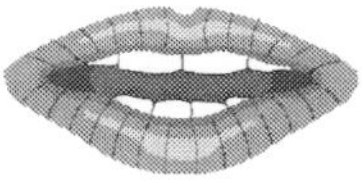

8. hopper

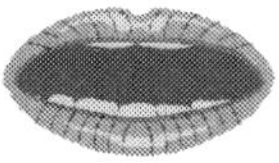

9. oriel

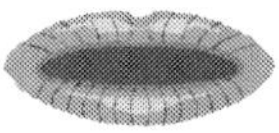

10. skylight

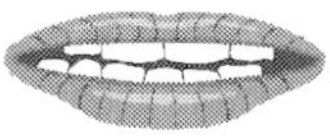

Lip-reading puzzle:

50. carpentry

The pictures below represent words to do with **woodworking** as a spoken list. The lip shape shown for each word is the first that would be seen by a lip-reader.

Here are the words as a written list:
Hammer, wood glue, saw, mallet, chisel, gauge, vice, clamp, compass, router.

Can you match the words on the list to the correct lip-shapes?

1.__________ 2.__________ 3.__________ 4.__________

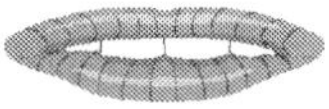
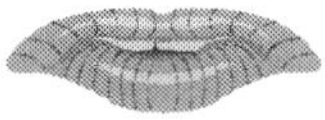
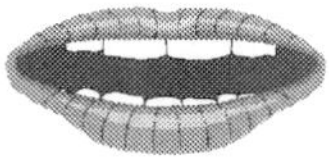
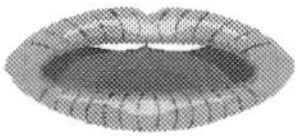

5.__________ 6.__________ 7.__________ 8.__________

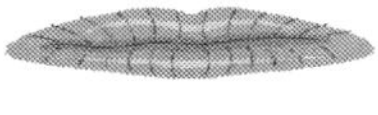
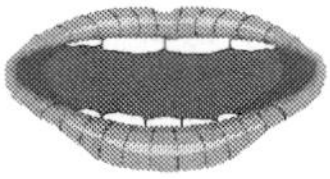
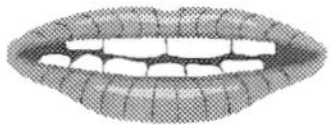
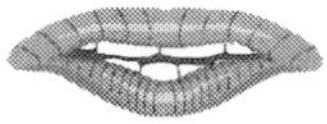

9.__________ 10.__________

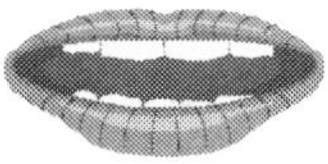
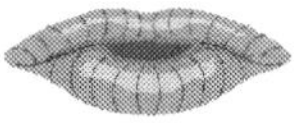

Solution:

50. carpentry

puzzle

The written list was:

Hammer, wood glue, saw, mallet, chisel, gauge, vice, clamp, compass, router.

The words can be matched to their respective initial lip-shapes in the following order.

1. vice

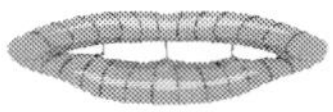

2. router

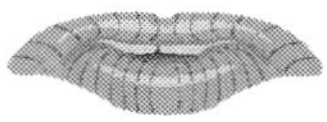

3. hammer

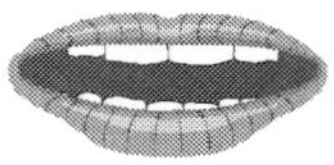

4. clamp

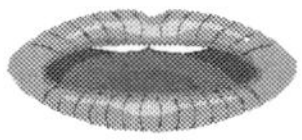

5. mallet

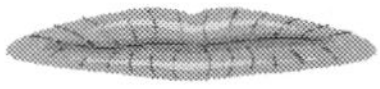

6. compass

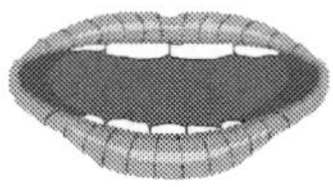

7. saw

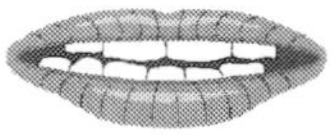

8. chisel

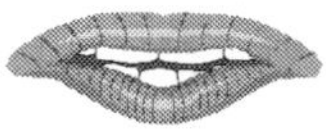

9. gauge

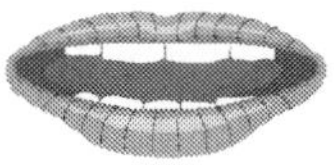

10. wood glue

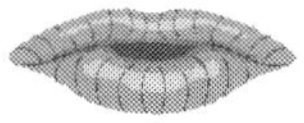

11.

12.

51. BASIC LIP-SHAPES

Lip shape A
for add, arch

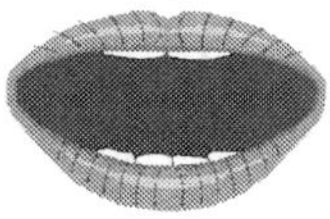

Lip shape E
for enter

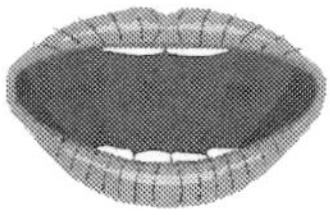

Lip shape EE
for even

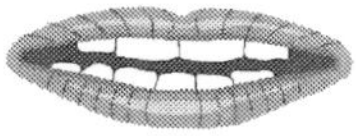

Lip shape ER
for urchin

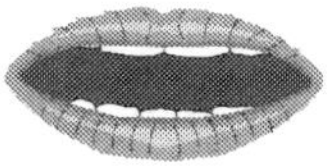

Lip shape I
for inner

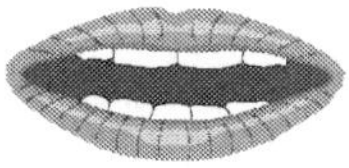

Lip shape J
for Junk

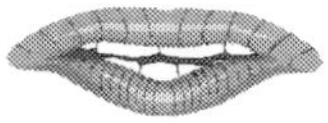

Lip shape K
for kite

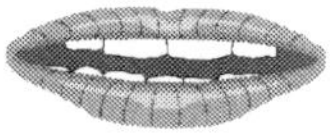

Lip shape L
for ladder

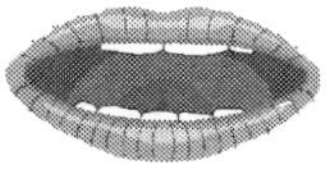

Lip shape M
ban, man, pan

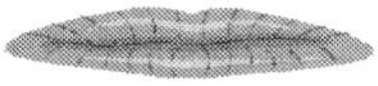

Lip shape O
for otter

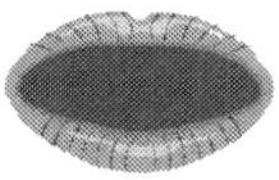

Lip shape OO
for ooze

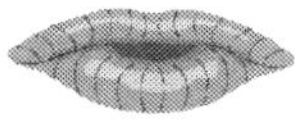

Lip shape R
for rabbit

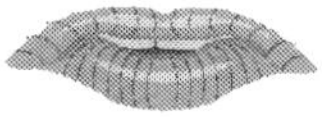

Lip shape S
for silent, zeal

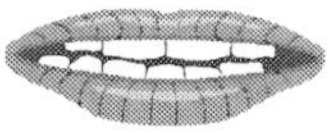

Lip shape T
for tent

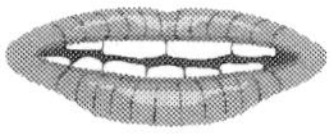

Lip shape TH
for thick, then

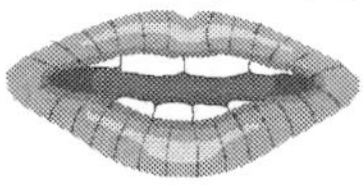

Lip shape U
for under

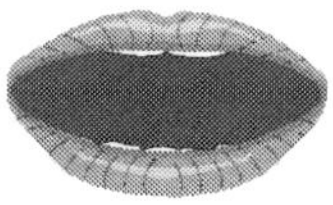

Lip shape UU
as in hood

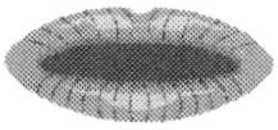

Lip shape V
for venture

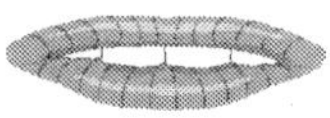

Lip shape W
for wisdom

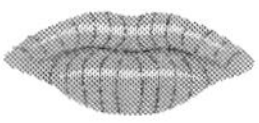

Lip shape Y
for unity, youth

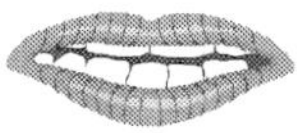

52. MODIFIED LIP-SHAPES

Some of the sounds in speech cannot be seen from the lips and are described by lip-readers as invisibles. This includes C, G, H and K sounds as in words like cool, gate, hook and kite. When we say these words, the C, G and H sounds are made while the lips are shaped to make the adjacent vowel sound. The lip-reader has to infer the presence of the C, G, H or K from the context.

Other groupings of sounds produce a modified single lip shape that contains elements of the lip-shapes of both sounds. The most notable of these are when C, G or H are preceded or followed by L, when C or G is preceded or followed by R, as in crow and cork. When L comes with EE or OO there is another compromised pair of lip shapes. Other examples are below.

Lip shape
K with L
for clue, clean
glance, glade

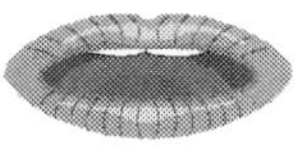

Lip shape
K with R
crack, grow
ground, crowd

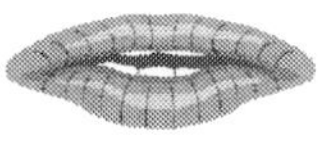

Lip shape
L with EE
for least, fleet
leak keel

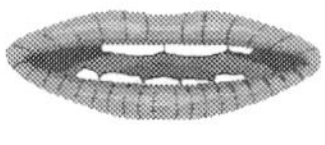

Lip shape
L with OO
for loot, blue
loose, cool

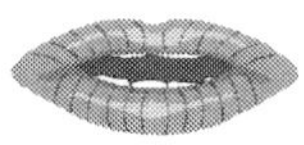

Lip shape
T with OO
for tool, lute

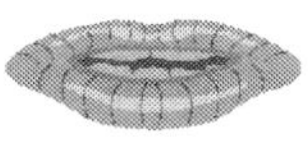

Lip shape
T with R
for trouble, treat

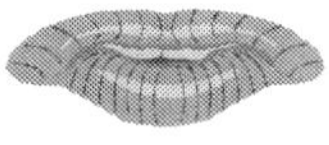

Lip shape
T with UU
for took,

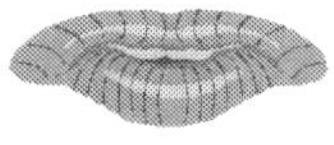

Lip shape
TH with R
for throw, thrill

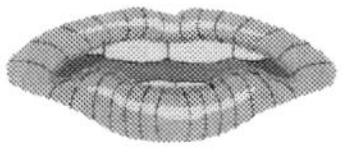

23344443R00063

Printed in Great Britain
by Amazon